The Mocha Manual to a Fabulous Pregnancy

The Mocha Manual to a Fabulous Pregnancy

Kimberly Seals-Allers

 Amistad *An Imprint of HarperCollinsPublishers*

THE MOCHA MANUAL TO A FABULOUS PREGNANCY. Copyright © 2006 by Kimberly Seals Allers. All rights reserved. Printed in the United States of America. No part of this book may be used or reproduced in any manner whatsoever without written permission except in the case of brief quotations embodied in critical articles and reviews. For information address HarperCollins Publishers, 10 East 53rd Street, New York, NY 10022.

HarperCollins books may be purchased for educational, business, or sales promotional use. For information please write: Special Markets Department, HarperCollins Publishers, 10 East 53rd Street, New York, NY 10022.

FIRST EDITION

Designed by Chris Welch
Illustrations by Raina Tinker

Library of Congress Cataloging-in-Publication Data

Allers, Kimberly Seals.
    The mocha manual to a fabulous pregnancy / Kimberly Seals-Allers.— 1st ed.
        p.   cm.
    ISBN-13: 978-0-06-076229-2
    ISBN-10: 0-06-076229-2 (pbk. :)
    1. Pregnancy—Popular works. II. African American women—Health and hygiene—Popular works. I. Title.
RG525.A55 2006
618.2'0089'96073—dc22   2005048098

08 09 10 BVG/RRD 10 9 8

For
Alma and James Seals,
Joseph, Kayla, and
Michael Jaden

Contents

FOREWORD   xi

1 *Great Expectations* PREPARING YOURSELF FOR THE
PREGNANCY JOURNEY   3

2 *The Pregnancy Lowdown* A TRIMESTER-BY-
TRIMESTER GUIDE   43

3 *Truth Versus Lies* THE REAL DEAL ON TEN COMMON
PREGNANCY MYTHS   83

4 *Pregnancy and Your Peeps* FROM YOUR GIRLFRIENDS TO YOUR PARTNER—YOUR RELATIONSHIPS ARE ABOUT TO CHANGE   97

5 *Not Your Ordinary Pregnancy* SINGLE MOTHER, HAVING TWINS, OVER AGE THIRTY-FIVE   117

6 *Seven Medical Conditions That More Commonly Affect Black Women and What to Do During Pregnancy*   141

7 *Managing Stress and the Strong Black Woman Syndrome in Pregnancy*   165

8 *The Darker Side of Pregnancy* DEPRESSION, LOSS, AND POSTABORTION PREGNANCIES   189

9 *Mocha Style* HOW TO LOOK LIKE A BABE WHEN YOU'RE HAVING ONE   217

10 *The Mocha Fix* SOLUTIONS FOR YOUR HAIR, SKIN, AND NAIL PROBLEMS   241

11 *Back for More* PREGNANCY THE SECOND TIME AROUND   251

12 *Mocha Money* THE NINE-MONTH GUIDE TO
FABULOUS FINANCES   259

ACKNOWLEDGMENTS   289

APPENDIX   293

INDEX   307

Foreword

Andrea Price-Rutty, M.D, F.A.C.O.G.

As long as I can remember, pregnancy, the process of bringing forth life, has held a particular fascination for me. On one hot August day, at the age of twenty-one, hopeful, starry-eyed, and full of excitement and enthusiasm than actual medical knowledge or common sense, when I was off from Case Western Reserve University it was nothing short of providential that my very first encounter with an actual living breathing patient two months into my medical school career would be a pregnant female. I will never forget this young woman—single, economically disadvantaged—and like myself was barely into her twenties. Unable to afford a private physician, she attended the prenatal clinic at the local University Hospital and afforded me the incredible privilege of sharing her pregnancy, the birth of her child, and her life. It was at this point that I knew I had to become an ob-gyn.

Eighteen years later, here I am, a seasoned ob-gyn practitioner having advised, examined, poked, prodded, hugged, cajoled, laughed, cried, encouraged, and harangued thousands of women of all ages, stages, races, and walks of life. I have cared for women in impoverished small towns, inner city settings, the rural Midwest, and wealthy East Coast suburbia. My medical mission work in poverty stricken Jamaica taught me how truly fortunate we are to live in a country where despite all its problems, even the least of us with some ingenuity, creativity, and persistence can obtain very good medical care.

Yet, in all my experience I remain intrigued, yet frustrated and saddened, by the disparate health care of women of color in general and of the unique needs of African American women in pregnancy in particular. But these needs are often overlooked and largely ignored. How can it be that in this day and age, in the most technologically advanced country on earth, that the infant mortality rate for African American babies is similar to that of some third world countries? Some of the disparity is a result of hereditary factors. For example, black women are more likely to suffer from hypertension and diabetes in pregnancy and, as a whole, tend to have smaller babies than our white counterparts. However, much of the disparity can be accounted for by socioeconomic factors, cultural factors, lack of information, and lack of access to the best medical care. By socioeconomic factors I mean that we are more likely to live in poverty which often means inadequate nutrition, an unhealthy living environment as well as suboptimal health at the time of conception. By cultural factors I mean we are more likely to be obese due to a diet high in starches and fats and lacking in fresh fruits and vegetables. As a people we often don't understand or value the concept of preventative health care and health maintenance and can't fathom going to see a doctor if we are not seriously ill. Lack of access means we don't often have health insurance and can't afford visits to the physician or prescription medications. Sometimes we lack basic transportation to get to medical facilities. The lack of information means that many of us don't know about some of the programs available to us to assist in overcoming many of above difficulties. We also often don't have basic medical information such as health screening tests that need to be performed on a regular basis.

Additionally, there are other things such as stress, community demands, and our eternal need as African American women to be all things for all people. We feel compelled to live up to the archetypal image of the strong black women, a born nurturer who ignores her own needs for the benefit of her family, friends, church, and coworkers. Even when we feel sick, tired, weak, or depressed, we are in denial about our need to be nurtured and taken care of. In general, we tend to have more on our plates which further exaggerates the typical emotional roller coaster of pregnancy. Add to that morning sickness, fatigue, back pain, swollen ankles, distress about weight gain, and a rapidly changing body and it is a wonder that we manage to emerge with body and soul intact. I have always maintained that if men were the ones having the babies they would get their epidural anesthesia the minute the pregnancy test turned positive and keep it flowing until the child turned twenty-one! Yet, through it all, our natural desire to be nurtured and taken care of remains our dirty little secret.

With so much experience, I thought pregnancy would be a piece of cake for me. It just goes to show you how wrong a sister can be! I was used to hearing stories about women who obsessed over urine pregnancy tests, fetal heartbeats, and every single ache and pain. But with my unlimited access to all things medical, I was able to take this pregnancy obsession thing to a whole "'nother level." I literally have pictures of my daughter, Chase, when she was nothing but a microscopic egg contained in a cyst on my ovary. I watched that cyst via ultrasound daily; until I was sure ovulation had taken place. I tell my patients to wait at least thirteen days after ovulation before taking a pregnancy test, yet seven days later I started taking one or two pregnancy tests daily to see if I was pregnant and my office manager couldn't understand why we kept running out of test kits. Fortunately several weeks into being pregnant I relaxed and was able to enjoy the experience of nurturing a life in my womb. After about week fourteen I even managed to stop watching the baby via ultrasound almost daily, mainly because I didn't want to slip up and accidentally reveal the sex, which I didn't want to know until birth. Even after very reassuring fetal testing results I still worried occasionally throughout the pregnancy about my "advanced maternal age" status (age thirty-five or older at the time of delivery). Even physicians have anxiety and moments of irrational behavior during pregnancy.

Meanwhile, my mother, who had given birth to six children herself and retired from nursing sometime around the dark ages, managed to completely ignore my medical license and forget my status as a board certified obstetrician, began giving me all sorts of well meaning but outdated advice. Despite my firm belief that the baby I was carrying was a girl, and the fact that I had always dismissed the myriad of superstitions and beliefs surrounding pregnancy as "old wives tales," when my seventh month rolled around and I was barely showing in front, but my butt had expanded threefold . . . I started to think that maybe my mother, my husband's psychic aunt, his eighty-seven-year-old grandmother, and the lady at the supermarket were all right—maybe I was having a boy.

It all culminated early one Friday morning when two days before my due date my water broke and I nearly missed my own delivery. At this point I always tell my patients to notify me immediately, but instead I grabbed a pair of XL Depends, my laptop, a handful of towels, and tried to head out to the office to finish some work. As I struggled to climb into my new mom-compatible SUV, my husband decided he had seen enough and dragged me back into the house by the sash of my hideous flowered maternity dress.

Not to be outdone by my mom who birthed six and my grandmother who birthed eight, I was determined to have a natural childbirth and all the bragging rights thereto appertaining.

From all my years on the Labor and Delivery floor I knew that the best way to accomplish this was to stay home and labor as long as possible. Initially my contractions were very irregular and mild. At this point I usually tell my patients to eat very lightly and nutritiously, rest between contractions, and save their strength for active labor. Yet I, the girl who will rewash and dry an entire load of clothes to avoid touching an iron, ironed all the babies' outfits, then unpacked and repacked my suitcase. When I got hungry I scarfed down a turkey club sandwich with bacon and cheese, some potato chips, and washed it all down with a diet Coke. Not exactly textbook medical protocol. I took a shower, posed for some last minute pictures of my pregnant self in what was soon to be the nursery, and took my time getting ready to leave for the hospital.

By now it was evening and the labor pains, while quite intense, were only coming every fifteen minutes and as long as I stayed on my feet and practiced the breathing techniques they were quite bearable. I always instruct all of my first time moms to wait until the pains are five minutes apart for at least an hour before coming into the hospital, but I never guessed that my own contractions would jump from fifteen minutes apart to every five minutes and then every two minutes all in the space of twenty minutes.

By the time we picked up my suitcase and headed for the door my pains were coming so fast and furious I could barely climb into the SUV. I tell my patients to leave plenty of time to get to the hospital, but here we were speed racing to the hospital doing fifty miles per hour down a side street. "Drive," I yelled between contractions. "If I deliver in this SUV I will never live it down." We made it to the hospital in record time and I hit the Labor and Delivery floor at a dead run, changed into my hospital gown at lightning speed, and barely made it to the hospital bed before a dutiful nurse reported sightings of a head. And while I tell my first time mothers to plan to push for two hours, it only took five minutes and three pushes before I was gazing into the eyes of Chase Noelle, my own personal miracle, feeling like the original Earth Mother, impossibly powerful, intensely womanly, and blessed by the Creator. Wow, I did it! Natural childbirth, and thanks to my

"Miss Know It All Obstetrician" attitude there was no time for blood work, paperwork, fetal monitors, or IVs. Heck, her head narrowly missed being born into a pair of XL Depends!

As I put my daughter to my breast for the first time and she latched on ravenously, sucking greedily like she knew what she was doing, I reflected on my own pregnancy experience which made one thing crystal clear. Unlike my newborn baby, who minutes after birth rooted instinctively—knowing exactly what to do at the breast—not even four years of medical school, four years of residency training, and nearly a decade of practicing obstetrics fully prepared me for this pregnancy business and all that it entails. Every pregnancy and birth experience is unique and there really is no standard pregnancy or delivery experience. Maybe there was a standard protocol back in the day when every pregnant mother in labor got an enema, was shaved bald, and had her butt sterilized in preparation for being knocked out with anesthesia so her baby could be pulled out with forceps. But thankfully in this era of modern obstetrics the pregnancy game has changed.

To put it simply, this is not your mother's pregnancy. The advent of new technology and an unprecedented explosion in medical knowledge over the past decade means that the field of obstetrics is continually growing and changing and improving. Now more than ever the wide spread availability of screening for chromosomal problems, genetic illnesses, fetal abnormalities, gestational diabetes, preterm labor, and hypertensive disorders of pregnancy to mention a few, combined with advancements in treatment of these conditions have made it even more crucial that all mocha mothers get early and consistent prenatal care. Never before has the chance of delivering a healthy full term infant been greater.

All this makes for a group of sisters who are in need of serious guidance. And not just the guidance that can come from stacks of pregnancy books, Web sites, prenatal classes, and even your obstetrician, but the kind of guidance, comfort, and support that only your sisterfriends can bring. That is what makes *The Mocha Manual to a Fabulous Pregnancy* so timely and unique. It gives expectant mothers the information they need most to thrive prepregnancy, in pregnancy, and beyond. Not only do you get the skinny on the most up-to-date medical information and advice, this book also lets you hear from everyday moms as well as celebrity moms on the issues most relevant to us sistergirls. Never before has there been a book by us, for us, that speaks directly to us . . . this is the real deal.

The way I see it, *The Mocha Manual* is an extremely important tool in reversing the statistical tide of low birth weight babies, preterm labor and delivery, and poor maternal and fetal outcomes so rampant in our communities. It doesn't matter if you are a highly educated corporate sister holding down the household with a six-figure income, if you have more in common with the aforementioned young single mom who inspired my entree into the obstetrical field, or like most of us, fall somewhere in between, this book reaches out across the ever widening chasm of culture and socioeconomic bias to provide black women with the same information and advantages that our majority sisters have enjoyed all along. This information empowers us as women to take control of our health and the health and lives of our unborn children. That is the most tangible way I can imagine of loving ourselves and ensuring the future of our African American community . . . and that is truly fabulous.

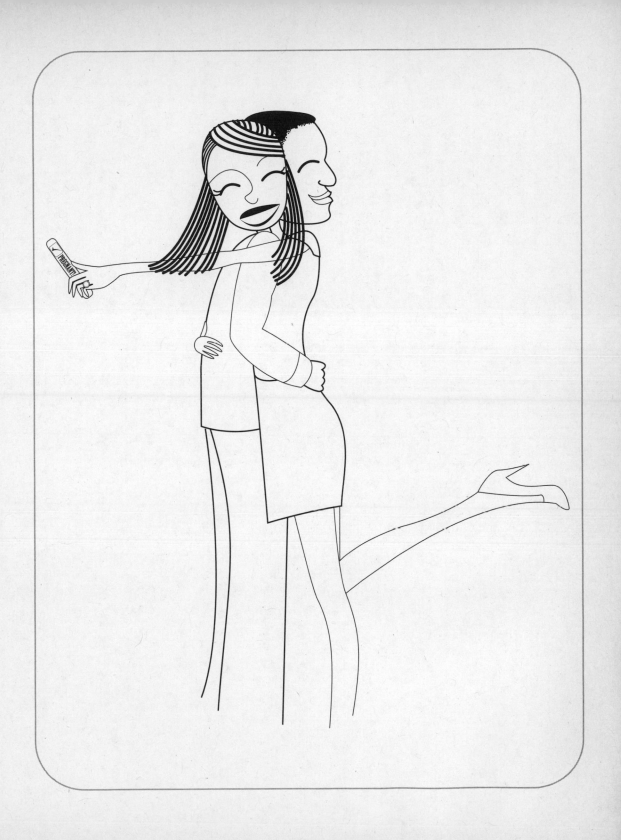

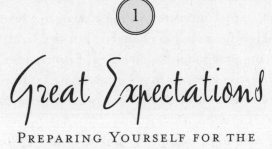

1

Great Expectations

PREPARING YOURSELF FOR THE
PREGNANCY JOURNEY

Congratulations! If you're reading this, that means you are either already pregnant or thinking about becoming pregnant. You know, expecting. With child. In the family way. Knocked up. Or as they said back in the day, the rabbit has died. However you label it, you are set to embark on a life-changing journey that will last roughly forty weeks and will allow you entrée into the exclusive sorority of motherhood, in which delivery is the ultimate hazing ritual. But what lies between then and now, between you now and you lying on a table with your legs cocked up, sweating, aching, and pushing like a grizzly bear, is the most awesome experience known to womankind. In fact, it is an odyssey so exhilarating in its exhaustiveness, so powerfully awe-inspiring and humbling, so life-transforming, that God knew that there wasn't even a slight chance that men could do the job. They can barely manage that toilet seat situation.

So here you are, a strong, beautiful black woman about to have a baby. Unfortunately, for most of us, this baby-making business has become more difficult than back in the days when our great-great-grandmamas squatted in the field, pushed out a youngin, and went back to picking cotton in the afternoon. And it's not that the baby-making formula has changed, but the "stuff" we have to deal with during pregnancy has changed. From career obligations, financial concerns, stress in the workplace, to family drama, girlfriend drama, husband or significant other drama—we have a lot with which to contend.

There are meetings, deadlines, spiritual and civic obligations, telephone check-ins on all the people who depend on you, and perhaps a robust social life. We're always on the go. We eat on the run and network on the go. For me, "downtime" is a quick visit to the bathroom. Nowadays that's when I open the mail. You probably feel the same way.

It's a common problem with black women. We are the original den mothers—always looking out for others, husbands, children, employers, family, and friends—while somehow managing to further our career, find a meaningful relationship, and keep our spirituality intact. We give up time for ourselves, to take care of others. We push ourselves even though we're either tired or the perennial "sick and tired," hungry, or in dire need of some me time. We do the Strong Black Woman thing convinced that strength, invincibility, suffering, and self-sacrifice define us as black women. This is part of our culture and upbringing. And it hasn't gone unnoticed.

From as early as the eighteenth century, researchers have commented on the dominance of women in slave communities. That notion has even led researchers to study the "carrying" role of black women as pillars in our community, serving as community workers, church mothers, and political agents of social change, to name a few roles. Even in song and poem, our literary light bearers like Nina Simone, Maya Angelou, and Zora Neale Hurston have referred to our ability to make a way out of no way. Heck, even Tupac rapped about it. But the fact remains, our double-duty, nurturing task of tending to family and community is very stressful, even with our creativity and indomitable spirit. The stereotype of the Strong Black Woman is a myth that creates unnecessary pressure and unrealistic expectations, and behind the façade of almost every typical strong woman are often pain and sorrow. We are notoriously good at tending to others but woefully bad at looking after ourselves. This poses a unique problem in pregnancy.

Your job for the next nine months is to do your personal best to bring a healthy child into the world. Pregnancy is a special time, a crucial time for you to focus on yourself and the life growing inside you. Particularly since black women, across all socioeconomic levels, still have the highest incidences of preterm labor and low-birth-weight babies. In fact, black women are 2.2 times more likely to have a low-birth-weight infant (under five and a half pounds) than their white counterparts. According to the Centers for Disease Control and Prevention (CDC), black women have a three to four times greater risk of a pregnancy-related death than white women. This is the largest racial gap in any of the maternal and child indicators that the CDC researches, and it has persisted for more than sixty years. We also have disproportionately high rates of premature births: 17.5 percent of all births to black women were premature in 2001, compared with a national average of 11.9 percent, according to the March of Dimes. And preterm birth is the leading cause of infant deaths in the United States. These numbers can't be ignored.

Understanding that the complexities of our lives as black women can influence our responses to various situations, including pregnancy, is key to helping us reverse the statistical tide in birth outcomes. So where does that leave you? Ready to exhale and let it go, I hope. Try to submit mentally to your body—reading and, this time, actually listening to its signals. Pregnancy is the perfect time to learn the art of surrender. Get out your white flag and start waving. Now, I'm no Iyanla, with all that let go and let God stuff, and the listening to the inner voice. Nor do I have forty principles that lead to spiritual strength and understanding. But I do strongly recommend taking a few moments for introspection. I'm pretty sure Iyanla would call it soul work. Take time daily to relax, breathe deeply, and concentrate on the new life growing (or soon to grow) inside you.

Let's start by taking a little personal inventory. What about your lifestyle? For example, do you often end up skipping meals? Or have you recently had a bag of microwave popcorn or a box of Oreos and called it dinner? Does the staff at your local fast food drive-through know you by name? Don't feel bad. Denene Millner, author of *The Sistah's Rules* and coauthor of the best-selling series What Brothers Think, What Sistahs Know and *The Vow: A Novel*, among others, admits that in her prepregnancy life she used to eat popcorn and sherbet for dinner most nights. Her refrigerator was always empty. As the pop culture reporter for a major New York daily newspaper, she spent most of her prepregnancy time at industry parties rubbing noses with celebrities. "There were many times when I would do interviews at midnight in the recording studio," Denene, now a mother of two, says. Pregnancy forced Denene to make some serious lifestyle changes and set some new healthy eating priorities.

Along with Denene, most of us don't have time to eat, yet alone eat healthfully. According to the American College of Obstetrics and Gynecology, pregnant women need to eat at least an extra three hundred calories each day—the basic equivalent of about two and a half cups of low-fat milk—for a daily total of between 2,100 and 2,500 calories. This doesn't sound too bad until you realize your regular recommended pregnancy diet is supposed to include ten extra grams of protein, nine servings of grains, three servings of fruit, and four servings of vegetables each day. When's the last time you had four servings of vegetables in one day?

Angelou Ezeilo, a mocha-colored attorney from West Orange, New Jersey, had a bad habit of skipping meals because of her hectic workday. She hated feeling guilty about not eating when she was pregnant but often found herself too busy (or so she thought) to eat. There are lots of specifics on pregnancy nutrition out there, but the main point now is to accept that most girls on the go have to make adjustments in their eating habits. Avoid sodium-laden processed and canned foods and salty foods, eat small meals frequently throughout the day, and try to eat organic foods whenever possible to prevent toxic chemicals from entering your system (see Appendix for pregnancy nutrition help). And be sure to wash all fruits and veggies thoroughly. "Never in my life have I thought so much about what I had ingested as I did when I was pregnant," says Kuae, from Montclair, New Jersey. Point number one in preparing for pregnancy changes; write it down: Eat better and frequently.

Point number two in preparing for pregnancy changes—and you might want to sit down for this one—is, Say good-bye to your body as you know it. If I had a dollar for every woman interviewed for this book who said she thought she would only get bigger in the stomach area, I'd have already bought my private island off the coast of Fiji. Your body will no longer behave the way it used to and it won't look the same either. Even you superexercising, Pilates, kick boxing, and spinning types should brace yourselves. But here's the great news. The most liberating (or pretty darn close) thing about pregnancy is that it is finally OK for your tummy to bulge. Liberate yourself from sucking it in all day. Get rid of the tummy-control-this, and spandex-microfiber-panel-that. Go on: stick it out.

Granted, for many this is easier said than done. We live in a very body-conscious world, not even including the state of matters in California. For many people, their body and perceptions of it play an integral part in their self-esteem and confidence. My girlfriend Charisse had been a size four since high school, and though she was elated at the thought of pregnancy, she struggled to accept her pregnant body. You see, she envisioned herself as the same size-four Charisse with just a lovely bump of baby growing in her midparts. But pregnancy is a total-body experience. Most women blow up all over, from those chubby cheeks to the water-retaining ankles. Those toned arms fill out a bit, and those once-tight thighs start to do the Harlem shake. And for many black women there is the dreaded and inevitable nose spreading and face ballooning. I'd be willing to testify in a court of law that somewhere around the end of my seventh month, some cruel yet stealthy intruder popped a needle into my face and hooked me up to a high-pressure air system. Move over, P. Diddy: I was the new Puffy! Back to Charisse—who was visibly depressed for a number of weeks that her pregnancy body expectations were dashed to pieces, and even more shamed at the depth of her body image issues. I'm thankful to say she got over it.

Even black women have issues about our body and weight gain. We used to classify it as a white woman's problem. Let's face it: we have always been known for our curvaceousness—ample thighs and hips, and the bigger the butt the better. That's our trademark and that's how our men like us, thankyouverymuch. Unlike in the white woman's world, not having a butt is a cause for shame and derision among black folks. But thanks to BET and Beyoncé, you now need to have a flat, washboard stomach, with a few curves below the waist. Fatty backs are a no-no, lower tummy pouches ain't cute, and I won't even start on spare tires. Black people have abandoned our healthy images of the Big Mamas we loved and the thick aunts who cradled us in their ample bosoms and have succumbed to a more mainstream ideology. Whether that is good or bad is not the subject of this book. But here's what's key: we all have body image issues. But pregnancy is no time for self-esteem issues tied to weight. It is completely inappropriate and selfish. If getting weighed at every doctor visit is a bit stressful, tell the nurse you don't want to know your weight unless there's a problem. Look the other way or stand on the scale backward. Regardless of what changes occur, remember that you are not the first weight-worrying mother, but your baby comes first. You are carrying a life, girl! Love your body!

Now that you've accepted that you will thicken a little, and quite possibly in places you'd rather not see more fat deposits, you should know that the recommended weight gain for a woman who began pregnancy at a normal weight is twenty-five to thirty-five pounds. If you begin pregnancy underweight, then you should gain twenty-eight to forty pounds, and if you're overweight, then your target weight gain is fifteen to twenty-five pounds. Your doctor can help you determine the weight gain that is right for you. But the general guidelines go something like this: four to six pounds in the first trimester, then average a pound a week in the second and third trimesters. Here's what I never read: gaining enough weight is especially important for black women since studies show that we have to gain more weight than white women in order to produce a baby of equal size. A hearty share of women I spoke to gained forty to fifty pounds, and some even lost weight in the first trimester.

If you can manage to change your thinking about making yourself a priority, eating healthfully, and being cool with your new voluptuousness, then you're halfway there. The other half is managing all the other physical and emotional changes your body will face over the next forty weeks. You can't control most of the physical changes, and when it comes to the hormonal changes, you're basically along for the ride. Here's a breakdown of some of what you can expect from your body and your emotions:

MORNING SICKNESS

Morning sickness is the standard by which all pregnancies are measured. If a woman complains of a difficult or miserable pregnancy, she likely had severe morning sickness. If a woman brags of her pregnancy glow and radiance, she probably didn't spend much of her first trimester poised in front of a toilet. Morning sickness can, in some cases, make or break a woman's opinion about this pregnancy business. But first, let's dispel two common myths:

First, morning sickness is a fat misnomer because it often lasts all day and can strike at any time. Second, morning sickness does not happen to every pregnant woman. In fact, studies show that only half of all expectant women get it. Morning sickness can run the gamut from occasional lightheadedness and dizzy spells, to full-fledged vomiting and nausea several times a day. Even the most severe morning sickness usually passes after the third month. There have been a lot of studies on the root cause of morning sickness with no definitive answers. Doctors know that the brain stem is the center of all the nausea and vomiting activity. But there are a number of theories about what causes this area to be overstimulated during pregnancy. Some probable causes include the high levels of hormones, the rapid stretching of the uterine muscles, a less efficient digestive system, the excess acid in the stomach, and a heightened sense of smell.

The one thing they do know for sure is that certain things such as stress and fatigue can make morning sickness worse. Unfortunately, there isn't a one-size-fits-all cure for morning sickness. In fact, there is no cure for morning sickness. Most women find relief through trial and error. Tracey from Saint Louis found that eating a piece of hard candy, a Jolly Ranchers or Starburst, just as she got out of bed did the trick. Others swear by ginger tea. Here are some more suggestions to try until you find what works for you:

1. Eat light and often, and do so before you get hungry. When your stomach is empty, it releases acids that can cause nausea. Carry snacks and bottled water with you at all times.
2. Don't rush in the morning. Rushing tends to aggravate nausea. Give yourself extra time to eat a few crackers, wait twenty minutes, and then get out of bed slowly and have breakfast.
3. Avoid tobacco smoke, which is known to increase morning sickness.
4. Avoid any sights, smells, or tastes that trigger queasiness.
5. Try Sea-Bands. These are one-inch bands, worn on both

wrists, that put pressure on the inner wrist and help alleviate nausea.

6. Acupuncture often works to relieve nausea.

BREASTS AND BEHIND

If you weren't given the ample breast gene or spent most of your young adult years quoting that "More than a mouthful is a waste" adage, then pregnancy may be your big score. Literally. The average woman gains two pounds in her chest, thanks to milk-producing glands that are starting to grow—and will continue to grow during pregnancy. Pretty soon you'll have breasts that enter a room at least thirty minutes before the rest of your body. "My boobs just kept getting bigger and bigger. I would just look at them and say, 'What the hell . . . ?'" says Mary, a plant supervisor from Detroit. The skin on your nipples and areola may also get a bit darker. Your partner will likely be all excited about this turn of events and may reason that this pregnancy thing isn't so bad after all. Of course, your breasts will also feel swollen and tender and generally hurt like the dickens for most of the first trimester—which means your partner may not be able to get close to your bodacious tatas for a little while. But enjoy them while you can.

Ariel, from Orange, Connecticut, was basically what you would call flat as a board. When she became pregnant, Girlfriend had more open blouses and plunging V-necks than Pamela Anderson. The bad news is, and as a sistah I must tell you, that the time will soon come when the size of your belly will dwarf even your Tyra Banks boobs. And while Ariel was the type who could go with just a camisole or without a bra at times, she quickly learned that this is not a good idea during pregnancy. Even you free-spirited Erykah Badu types need to buy a good support bra. Trust me: with all the stretching, swelling, and future sucking that's about to go on, this is the time to give your new milk jugs some serious TLC.

Of course, with the euphoric state of a buxom chest comes this sobering news: Your breasts will probably never be the same again. Once they've been stretched, and remain that way until after you're done nursing, the skin never fully retracts to its previous tight form. Some women are nervous about breast-feeding because of what it will do to their breasts. Trust me: pregnancy alone will change your breasts, so, if you can, you might as well give your child the best start by breast-feeding.

This brings me to the butt. With all the expanding parts in front of me, I never really checked out what was going on in the back, until one day, I happened to take a slow stroll past the mirror. My hips were wider and my butt was spreading like jam and looking more rounded than ever before. The traditional explanation is that nature wants to ensure that the fetus won't starve, so your body packs up extra food supplies in the form of fat on your hips, butt, and other places. Whatever the rationale, remember this: even if you thought your butt could get no bigger, pregnancy may surprise you, and always check the rear view when you're trying on maternity gear!

All of this talk about the derriere brings us to a most sensitive topic among the ladies: underwear. Now I was convinced I'd wear my thong all the way into the delivery room. Even while I was blowing up like a float in the Macy's parade, I was hanging on to the thong. I was resolved *not* to do the granny panties thing. I was painfully squeezing myself into the thing, wriggling every morning, determined to feel sexy underneath regardless of the situation in my growing midparts. I didn't listen to my body, but my stomach was so big it was rejecting the thong. My body was shouting NO!! with a bullhorn. But I'd just pull the thong up. My big stomach would roll it right back down. I'd pull it back up, and it would roll right back down. One day my husband witnessed this battle between bulge and a spandex blend, this war between fetus and fabric, and said, "Babe, why don't you get some comfortable panties?" After I went off on a pregnancy-hormone-induced tirade about how he couldn't understand how important it was for me to hold on to something from my former self, to feel sexy and still have some aspect that was still ME!!!, I decided to lie down and sleep on it. Plus, I had tired myself out trying to get them on. I tried to sleep, but the dern thong was cutting off my circulation around where the thigh meets the pelvis area, and I couldn't get comfortable. In fact, it was really starting to hurt. But I couldn't get them off by myself. I now screamed to my husband to help me. Get scissors, a chain saw, the jaws of life; I don't care: just get these things off me. He had to cut the thong to free me, and he couldn't do it fast enough as far as I was concerned. I did wear a pair of thongs one more time—on the way to the department store for some ultrasoft, cotton granny panties. And let me tell you, ladies, once you've experienced the comfort of extralarge cotton underwear, you will never look back!! So don't be afraid to cross over. Nobody is checking you for VPL (visible panty lines) when you're pregnant. And you'll have enough discomforts without adding a piece of fabric piercing the middle of your butt to the list. Now that you can't wear belts or shirts that need to be tucked in, you'll have a lot more available drawer space for your big bloomers, anyway. Trust me. Be comfortable.

Hair and Nails

Thanks to amped-up hormones that boost metabolism and circulation, your skin cells are well fed during pregnancy. As a result, most women find their hair grows faster and/or thickens beautifully during pregnancy. Unfortunately, some women have a lot of shedding and hair loss after delivery, when hormone levels drop back to normal.

The downside to all this increased hair growth is that the growth is not limited to your head. Pregnancy-induced hirsutism, or excessive hair growth in women, most commonly strikes the facial areas (lips, chin, and cheeks) but can also affect the legs, arms, back, and belly. Kaia, from Bowie, Maryland, isn't the only woman who said her vaginal hair also grew thick. My armpits looked like I had Buckwheat in a headlock. This can be one area where pregnancy becomes more high maintenance than you imagined because you can spend more time shaving and getting waxed. Diane, from Columbia, South Carolina, had to get a lip and chin wax every week.

Your nails are another beneficiary of all the increased protein and vitamins going on in your body. They will be longer and firmer, and if yours are breaking off or brittle, then you should discuss that with your doctor because it may be a sign that you are not getting enough nutrients to support you and your baby properly. Consider this a good time for pampering yourself with more manicures and pedicures.

Gums

You may notice that your gums bleed when you brush your teeth. Can't remember the last time you visited the dentist? You could have a periodontal disease called *pregnancy gingivitis*, which occurs when elevated hormone levels cause the blood vessels in your mouth to expand or swell. Don't take bleeding gums lightly. There's evidence that severe periodontal disease may increase your risk of having a preterm or low-birth-weight baby. To keep the situation in check, floss regularly, make an appointment for your six-month dental checkup, and call your dentist immediately if you suspect you have an infection. It's also just good sense to brush and floss more, especially at night. I had a habit of waking up hungry at about 3:00 A.M. or so. I thought I was being a good mommy-to-be by eating lots of fruits and going back to bed. A few months down the road, a gnawing pain in my teeth sent me to the dentist, who said I had cavities. What! I hadn't had cavities since my teen years. I'm not a candy, chocolate, or sugary-drink kind of person, either. The dentist said that the natural sugars in fruits were the culprit, and that not brushing after those twilight fruit binges had likely led to these cavities. So don't say I didn't warn you.

Gas

There's really no cute way to say this: pregnancy involves a lot of farting and burping. It's not your fault, but those hormones slow down the digestive process. Your food sits in your stomach a lot longer than usual because your sluggish digestive system isn't moving things along as quickly as before. "All of a sudden I started burping all the time. Even my husband said, 'What's up with you and all this burping?' It started even before I missed my period. But that was my sign. I was pregnant," says Tracey, of Saint Louis, Missouri.

That means you can have the kind of farts and burps that melt paint off the walls, send young children running for air, and make your husband's releases look like a rookie effort. This may not be so bad when you're home and you can just laugh it off or give the sheets a few good fluffs. As I told my husband, inhaling my gaseous fumes, no matter how toxic, was the least he could do in this alleged "joint effort" to bring forth a child. But when you're at work in an important meeting, in the confined space of your office, or in line at the grocery store with other unsuspecting patrons, the gas problem can bring on a lot of anxiety. You can always try to make a mad dash to the ladies' room just as you feel things start to percolate (hoping that it's empty when you arrive), but in my experience you rarely make it there in time. I kept a small perfume spray in my office and another in my purse and would discreetly spray after a bomb detonated. But, between us gals, I'm really not sure it helped much.

Stretch Marks

Let's face it: there's a whole lot of stretching going on during a pregnancy. And since there have never been any reports of a woman just bursting at the seams, we know the skin has amazing elasticity. But not without consequences. This brings us to the dreaded stretch marks. In darker-skinned women they appear as dark streaks; for women with lighter skin, stretch marks are lighter. Interestingly, stretch marks are less common in black women than in women of other races. But our skin tends to lose elasticity faster, resulting in loose skin and fat pouches around the stomach, thighs, butt, and hips. Now the experts will tell you that there's nothing you can do to prevent stretch marks. They say there is no foolproof method of preventing them, and it totally depends on genetics. Perhaps. But most women won't go down without a fight. Patrice, from Fresno, California, greased up at least twice a day cocoa butter, shea butter, olive oil, you name it, she tried it. Patrice swears she defied genetics because although her mother has stretch marks, she does not. You have to make your own call. Keep in mind that these lotions also help relieve the constant itching that comes with a stretched belly. The itching is something no one can explain to you, except to say that at times I was sure this is what it must feel like to have fleas. If you are really suffering, there are creams and antihistamines available from your doctor to help avoid ripping yourself to shreds. Some women get an extremely itchy rash that covers the abdomen, butt, and thighs after the thirty-fifth week of pregnancy. The rash isn't harmful to your baby and will go away after you deliver.

CONSTIPATION

You may also experience constipation. The medical books will tell you that all the extra hormones that are produced during pregnancy cause the intestine to relax, digest more slowly, and become less efficient. The hormones make your bowels more relaxed, too, so elimination is more sluggish. To help get matters moving, eat plenty of fruit, fiber, vegetables, and whole grains, and drink as much water as you can. Many women say a brisk walk every day helped keep them regular. Prolonged constipation can often lead to . . .

Hemorrhoids

Hemorrhoids, or piles, are varicose veins of the rectum that pop out of your derriere. They can cause itching, pain, and rectal bleeding. Like I said, there's no gingerly way to put this. But between 20 and 50 percent of all pregnant women are hit with hemorrhoids. Some women also get fissures, cracks in the anus caused by constipation. They can appear with hemorrhoids or on their own, and they are extremely painful. The key to avoiding hemorrhoids or other anal maladies is keeping constipation at bay. If you feel blocked up, ask your doctor to recommend a stool softener (only get one he recommends). If hemorrhoids do strike, avoid pressure on the rectal veins by sleeping on your side, not your back. Don't strain when having a bowel movement. A cotton pad soaked with witch hazel or ice packs applied directly to the area may also help.

If you are having excruciating pain in that area but can't spot a hemorrhoid, run to your doctor. It could be an anal fissure, which, after having experienced one, I can tell you must translate into Latin for the most intense, torturous pain known to humans. If you are so unlucky, you will likely end up where I did, at the proctologist, aka the butt doctor. So let me prepare you. My first visit to the proctologist revealed one glaring truth: no one under the age of eighty visits these guys. So there I was in the waiting room with the entire cast from the movie *Cocoon* with canes and walkers in tow. It was pretty embarrassing, but that was nothing compared to the actual examination. The diagnosis was horrific. I had a fissure—a tiny tear in my butthole. I couldn't believe it. The good news about fissures is that they can heal within a few days if you can keep your stools soft. Increase your intake of dietary fiber and drink plenty of water. Your doctor may also recommend an analgesic cream (never use without your doctor's okay) and warm bath soaks. The moral of this story is, try to prevent constipation in the first place to avoid them.

LEG CRAMPS

Leg cramps, which occur mainly at night, are particularly common in the second and third trimesters. It is believed some leg cramps are caused by too much phosphorus and too little calcium circulating in the blood. Some doctors say a calcium supplement that doesn't contain phosphorus may be the key. Others say that eating something salty before you go to bed may make the cramps disappear, or that a magnesium supplement may reduce the cramps. Denise from Manassus, Virginia, swears by eating a banana every day to get rid of leg cramps. Older relatives and her girlfriends said it's the potassium in bananas, and it worked for her. Run it past your doctor and see what she says, before taking any medicine or vitamin supplements. Here are some other helpful tips: Don't curl your toes. Don't make the bed up so tightly that the weight of the bedding presses down on your toes. Elevate your feet above heart level, to help circulation. If you find yourself screaming for the Lord in midcramp, ask your partner to grip your heel, and, using a forearm, push your foot up while holding the knee straight with the other hand. If you can bear someone touching that area, try lightly massaging the cramped area with a little oil or lotion. If nothing brings you relief, contact your doctor to rule out the slight possibility that a blood clot developed in the vein.

RUNNY NOSE/NASAL CONGESTION

Feeling stuffed up? About 30 percent of women get nasal congestion without any other cold symptoms during pregnancy. For some it lasts the entire pregnancy; for others this feeling occurs in the last few months. Don't worry; it's just another fabulous by-product of all those amped-up hormones that cause swelling in the mucous membranes lining the nose and may even make you produce more mucus. What's more, your blood volume pumps up by about 40 percent during pregnancy and your blood vessels expand to create space for all that extra fluid. This can lead to swollen nasal membranes as well.

If you have nasal congestion along with other coldlike symptoms such as coughing, sneezing, sore throat, or mild aches and pains, you probably have a cold. Colds are common during pregnancy because your immune system is weakened and you're more vulnerable to infections. Speak to your doctor about any possible cold remedies you can take (be warned: the list is very short).

Otherwise, steam on its own can be a good remedy for nasal congestion. Take a warm shower before bed, or use a vaporizer or humidifier to add more moisture to the air in your room. Of course, the old-school method of a pot of boiling water in the room works, too. You can also try sniffing some eucalyptus oil on a cotton ball or some saline drops. If you don't get much relief, take comfort in knowing that congestion usually clears up a few days after delivery.

Spider Veins/Varicose Veins

Varicose veins are basically swollen blood vessels that develop or get worse during pregnancy. What's behind it? The valves that send the blood through the veins back to the heart soften in pregnancy, and sometimes they don't send the right amount of blood through the legs. That leads to collecting of blood and swelling of the veins. They can also be caused by your increased blood volume or an expanding uterus that puts pressure on the veins that carry blood from the lower limbs to the heart. Either way, varicose veins can be painful or just unsightly. A family history or being overweight can also contribute to the condition. To prevent or minimize varicose veins during pregnancy, avoid standing for a long time or sitting with legs crossed.

＊ Keep your feet and legs elevated whenever possible. A stool or box under your desk can do the trick at work, and you can put your feet up on a pillow when lying down at home.

* Sleep on your left side with your feet on a pillow. There's a large vein on the right side of your body called the *inferior vena cava*. Lying on your left side relieves it of the weight of the uterus and lessens the pressure on the veins in the lower limbs.
* You may be advised to get those prescription-strength stockings, better known as graduated compression stockings. They do a great job of supporting your legs and preventing your varicose veins from getting any worse, but they haven't been spotted in tones that flatter, complement, or vaguely resemble black skin tones. If you must wear them, put them on before getting out of bed in the morning. They are usually tight at the ankle and get looser as they go up the leg. This design prevents blood from collecting in the calves and supports surface veins.

LINEA NIGRA

You've probably heard about a dark line that appears down the middle of your tummy from the navel down, where the rectus muscle is stretched. Just as the pregnancy hormones make your nipples darker, they also darken a line that runs from the center of your abdomen to the top of your pubic bone. You probably never noticed this line until pregnancy. But it will fade within weeks or months after delivery.

VAGINAL DISCHARGE

Your vagina is going through a number of changes, and you may have an unusual discharge. A thin, mild-smelling discharge called *leucorrhea* is normal during pregnancy. As your pregnancy progresses, the discharge may increase and become quite heavy. You may want to try wearing a panty liner. Never use a tampon, which can introduce unwanted germs into the vagina. The change in odor and taste may put off your partner from any visits "downtown," but the discharge itself is nothing to worry about. It is important to keep the area dry and clean, and to avoid deodorant soaps, perfumes, or other irritants. If you develop a discharge that is greenish or yellowish, is thick, has a foul odor, and is accompanied by itching, burning, or soreness, you should consult your doctor to rule out any possible infection.

Another change in the vagina is that the glands that secrete oil in your vulva increase in activity. These glands can get infected if they are blocked by dead skin or a blackhead. Since a lot of black women have supercurly pubic hair, some may get hair bumps from the hairs curling underneath the skin. In some cases, the hair bumps become infected and turn into an abscess. If this happens, never squeeze it. That will only make it worse. Try warm compresses and try to keep the area clean and dry at all times. Wear breathable cotton panties, which also help absorb moisture. If the abscess does not seem to be improving, go to your doctor.

While we're on the vagina, a lot of women obsess about the stretching of the vagina after the childbirth thing. There are lots of urban legends out there about the husband who complained that the stuff wasn't as tight anymore after the birth. Or how the vagina now feels like an oversized jacket instead of tight-fitting glove. I've never met one woman who actually said this is true. Of course, most men are so happy to get some after being on the bench for such a long time, they probably wouldn't even have noticed. If you're really worried about things getting stretched out of shape, do Kegel exercises. Contract the same muscle that you would use to stop your pee-pee midstream ten times a day. But I'm pretty sure you'd have to deliver the entire Wayans family in one shot to do some real damage.

SEX

Since we're in that region, let's talk about sex. You may feel that sex is one area where you need no advice. It is, after all, how you got into this mess. But even the hottest mama will find that sex and pregnancy make a strange mix. Medically, your body is giving all the go-ahead signs. When pregnant, your labia enlarges because it is engorged with blood—the same type of physical reaction as sexual arousal. Whoa, talk about pregnancy perk number one. Lots of women report deeper and longer-lasting orgasms when pregnant, and most found new joy in taking a brisk walk, if you know what I mean. Your body is definitely ready. But the other component of sex for most women is emotional. And with pregnancy, emotions are erratic to say the least. Most of us ladies are all about the mood. There's nothing worse than being in the mood and your man says something stupid to kill it. But remember those pregnancy moods are fast and furious and can turn on a dime—you can be thinking about being with your man all day, scheming a way to jump his bones when he gets home from work. But let him walk through the door, not mention how sexy you look in his favorite nightie (which is now stretched beyond recognition across your bigger body), and Mount Saint Weepy erupts with a fury. The moment is definitely over, and you can't recover the way you used to. One minute you want it bad *now!*; the next, if your husband gets within five feet of you, he's in danger of losing a limb.

You may also have a tough time emotionally adjusting to your new body, and that may affect the way you feel sexually. Lots of women said they did not feel sexy when pregnant, even though their husband was turned on by their pregnant state. After surveying tons of women, I found roughly three reactions to sex during pregnancy: Either it brings out your va-va-va voom and increases your interest in sex, or you can't be bothered at all, or—the most confusing one for the man—your drive rides up and down, no pun intended. As luck would have it, many times your partner is having the exact opposite reaction. "My husband thought I was really sexy and he was all was over me all the time, and I was like, 'Dude, I'm sore; please back up off me,' " says Kareen, from Philadelphia, Pennsylvania. Some women who had absolutely no desire for sex still felt obligated to lie down and take one for the team every now and then—you know how men can get when they don't get their "medicine"—and then get right back to reading their baby books.

There may be some situations when your doctor may actually

recommend abstaining from sex. These circumstances may include any time there is unexplained bleeding, during the first trimester if you have a history of miscarriage or there are signs of possible miscarriage, or in the last eight to twelve weeks if you have a history of premature labor or are having signs of premature labor. At other times, let common sense be your guide. As my doctor told me, "If it hurts, don't do it." Or at least hold off until you get some clarity from your physician.

Even if you have the go-ahead, the first trimester can be particularly tough. Extreme tiredness, nausea, vomiting, really sore boobs—not exactly the kind of stuff that puts a girl in the mood. This is a really good time to teach your man an important lesson about pregnancy (there's more on your man and pregnancy in Chapter Four). Times when you're too tired, sore, or engrossed in baby books to have an interest in sex are not a reflection of your love for him, his sexual prowess, or the way you feel about Mr. _____ (enter pet name for penis here). You may have to keep reassuring him about this one.

By your second trimester, you may start getting your groove back, now that the pesky vomiting has subsided. By then, however, your body has probably changed a lot. Your old faithful moves and surefire favorite spot might not be so easy to find with more tummy, thighs, hips, and whatnot thrown into the mix. And it will take you longer to reach orgasm. But be assured, those who put in the extra work to find (and wait for) the new path to climax are graciously rewarded with superintense pregnancy orgasms.

Another sexual plus is that you're already pregnant. Not having to worry about failed birth control or about birth control at all, for that matter, can be very liberating. Sex during pregnancy brings about a certain freeness and relief; after all, the deed is done, so just let 'er rip. I don't have to tell you that as your stomach grows, the missionary position is out, so experiment with different rear-entry or standing positions. It may take a while to find a position that is comfortable, but, hey, that's the fun part!

There is one issue, however, that every man, at some point, will worry or express concern about. Many men have a fear that by having sex they may somehow harm the baby. This is just another insane by-product of men's obsession with penis size, and the typical arrogance of a man to assume that *his* penis is the one so large it can actually reach that far. Never in history has an unsuspecting fetus been poked in the head by a penis. But the worry freaks out a lot of men. "My husband was afraid he would hurt the baby," says Kim from Jacksonville, Florida. "I know that's the biggest myth in the world, but I couldn't really be bothered anyway so I just left it alone." Some men won't have intercourse with their wife for the whole nine months (although they still expect other services, if you know what I mean), and other men say they were too cautious to enjoy themselves fully. This is a good time for open communication and a diagram. Show him a magazine or book that illustrates the baby and all of its protective fluids and sacs. This may help rest his concerns. If not, enjoy this time off; you'll be back in the cut soon enough.

Urination

Even from when your baby is no bigger than a lima bean, you will have to pee-pee all the time. Your uterus is expanding and the extra hormones contribute to the problem. You'll probably have to tinkle during the night at least once or twice. The situation only gets worse at the very end of your pregnancy, when the baby has crept down into your pelvis. I think getting up all night to pee is also nature's way of preparing you for those middle-of-the-night feedings and crying spells in the months to come. If you're lucky, you may also find that you're able to get up, pee, rinse your hands, and doddle back into the bed without really waking up.

The need to urinate also becomes extremely urgent rather quickly. One minute you sense a need to go, and seconds later you have to pee right NOW! This is one of the many things most men don't get about pregnancy. So if your partner is driving and disregards your urgent need to go, simply remind him how much it will cost to clean his nice leather seats. This one always works.

The other problem with peeing during pregnancy is that you have to pee on demand a lot. Everytime you turn around, somebody is asking you to pee in a cup. If you want to impress me, don't tell me you endured forty hours of labor with no pain medication. Tell me you have the dexterity to pee in a two-inch-diameter cup over and over again without messing up your hands—a real test of skill when you're large and wobbly and can't even see your vagina anymore. If you're that woman, I've got a bottle of Dom Perignon waiting for you.

A cautionary note: Sometimes a cough, sneeze, or laugh can make it leak out on its own, without your being able to control it. My friend Raquel had that problem. It didn't help that her husband is a constant jokester. She wore a panty liner during the whole pregnancy.

Clumsiness

Ramped-up hormones, looser joints, and a new body to navigate can lead to a bad case of the clumsies. Don't feel bad if you're dropping things all the time, tripping over your own feet, or losing your balance often. You're carrying more weight, your center of gravity has changed now that your uterus is expanded, and your fingers, toes, and other joints are loosened by increased hormones. Things get worse in the last trimester but will ease up after delivery. In the meantime, avoid situations that require dexterity, like climbing stadium stairs and dancing on tables. Watch out for wet, icy surfaces, and don't be embarrassed to grab those handrails and take it slow. If you should fall, contact your doctor immediately. Your baby is pretty well protected in its sac, but check in to make sure everything is okay.

If, for some reason, your clumsiness is combined with blurred vision and lightheadedness, call your doctor immediately. This could be a sign of an inner ear infection, or a virus, so get it checked out.

Acne and Rashes

While there's lots of talk of the pregnancy glow, radiant skin and the rest, there are those women whose increased hormones produce another reaction—acne. This can bring on all the anxiety of puberty. And there's not much you can do (see Chapter Ten for more on skin care), but take comfort in knowing that this too shall pass.

Then there's that thing called the "mask of pregnancy." I always hated that expression because it makes it sound all mysterious like the mask of Zorro, when really it's an ugly darkened blotch or, worse, blotches on your face. The cause are those hormones again. Some women have found a thicker foundation covered it, but that didn't work for others. Do remember this: exposure to sunlight makes it worse. Facial blotches can be one of the more distressing pregnancy maladies, but they will disappear after the baby is born.

Moles

Lots of black women have more mole activity. It's always been another one of my telltale signs. They tend to pop up around the neck and shoulders. Also, moles that were essentially beauty marks turn into full-fledged protruding growths. Most will disappear after delivery. With me, after each pregnancy, one or two stick around for the after party.

Your Brain

Sure you're smart, and always will be. But during pregnancy there will be many times when you will both need reassurance and need to reassure others of this fact. That's because research shows that women in their second to third trimester have a significant decline in memory, known among other moms-to-be as "pregnancy brain." This basically means utter forgetfulness and lack of logical thinking. Ask my coworker, Cora, about how during my second pregnancy, I would just forget what I was saying right in the middle of my own sentence. If and when this happens to you, take solace in knowing that other women have experienced the same thing.

HORMONES AND EMOTIONS

Pregnancy brain is closely related to pregnancy madness, which acts a lot like a volatile mix of Alzheimer's disease, premenstrual syndrome (PMS), and, as they say, going postal. If you think this doesn't apply to you, remember that crazy people generally don't think they are crazy. As Tina from Houston, Texas, puts it, "When the hormones hit you, they really hit you. The emotional ride is unbelievable." Sometimes I would cry for no known reason. "One time I cried because we were out of mayonnaise, and I had my mind set on a tuna fish sandwich," says Patricia from Albany, New York. I'm not making this stuff up. Other women report crying over diaper commercials, cute baby clothes, and missed parking spaces. There were times when I knew at first why I started crying, but then I forgot what the reason was. The other thing about your emotions is that they can change very quickly and dramatically, or you may feel things that just don't make any sense. "Just the sight of my husband made me feel like, 'I hate him,' but I didn't know why," says Tia, from Saint Louis. This may all sound utterly ridiculous, but you'll remember these words soon enough. Please don't believe anyone who tells you that pregnancy was the most emotionally fulfilling and stable time of her life. I guarantee you she is lying.

DREAMS

Nobody knows why, but during pregnancy you will dream some of the most outlandish, completely ridiculous, vivid dreams. I've had dreams about romantic interludes with a boss I hated and being butt naked in Penn Station with a cow chasing me. Then you have typical dreams about falling, drowning, swimming, or delving into caves, which most dream experts say have to do with increased feelings of vulnerability. According to dream readers, deep swimming or going into caves is related to going deep inside oneself to prepare for birth, and dreaming of animals is about bonding with your baby in an instinctive or animal-like way.

Others dreams aren't so deep. "Whatever I last watched on TV, I dreamed about it. I had to stop watching shows like *ER* and *Law & Order*, and I couldn't even watch the news. It got so bad I had to limit myself to, like, the Food Network at night," says Lorraine from Mableton, Georgia. If you can, keep a dream journal. If nothing else, it will be good for a hearty laugh down the road.

CRAVINGS

The sense of urgency becomes particularly acute when dealing with cravings. These are uncontrollable, strong desires for strange and varied foods, drinks, cookies, spices, snacks, ice cream, or any combination thereof. Some cravings are really specific: my friend Ivy from Saint Louis craved Sonic chili dogs with everything on them and a root beer soda every day, while other women craved spicy foods, or anything dairy. I love Italian food. During my first pregnancy, I had to have a mozzarella and tomato salad drizzled with olive oil and balsamic vinegar almost every day—not a cheap craving. On my off days, I needed Taco Bell. Go figure. The fact is that cravings make absolutely no sense. "In the first half of my pregnancy, I craved sour. Sour Blow Pops, sour worms, and stuff like that," says Lorraine, from Mableton, Georgia. "Then it flipped to sweet—pink lemonade, and Shirley Temples." Denise from Manassus, Virginia, had a thing for soft serve ice cream shakes. "This place near my house has fifteen flavors and every day I'd try a different one and then start all over again." Cravings can appear right after you've had what appears to everyone around you to have been a perfectly satisfying meal. Inevitably, at some point in your pregnancy your partner will say the most ridiculously asinine, completely inappropriate comment, like "But you just ate." Or, "Are you going to eat another bag of Oreos?" When this happens—and I'm warning you that even the most Kenny Latimore–Musiq Soulchildesque, romantically sensitive brother will do it—please remember to do your part to stop black-on-black crime. Resist the urge to knock him upside the head with your purse, baby book, cell phone, bag of chips, or whatever is in your reach. Remember it's a pregnancy thing—they don't understand.

Phew! Reading all of that may have been pretty traumatizing. But remember that the beauty and the curse of pregnancy is that nobody can tell you exactly how it will be for *you*. In fact, some women get every possible pregnancy by-product and then some. Others don't get any of the distressing ailments. They just sail through pregnancy with no morning sickness, no constipation, beautiful skin, and only one untimely fart. That's what makes the journey so amazing. That's why you will soon want to talk to every woman who's ever been pregnant: to hear about her journey. Just a word of caution here: There is something known as too much information on pregnancy. I know that sounds strange because most of us are information-overloading, overanalyzing, give-me-the-nitty-gritty-details-and-don't-leave-anything-out kind of girls. But please trust me on this one. Know your threshold for too much information (TMI). I never wanted to watch those up-in-the-vagina birthing videos or the C-sections on TV. I figured that if I knew everything that was going on down there and had the visuals to go with it, there was a good chance I'd chicken out, freak out, or pass out. I don't even know how anyone could agree to those coochie cams anyway. My sense of obligation to educate humanity on the realities of childbirth is not that strong. And quite frankly, if God wanted women to see it all, he would have given us some sort of Go-Go Inspector Gadget extendable neck option, so we could crank up a few extra inches of vertebrae just to check it all out. But he didn't. And I take that as a divine sign. Now, your husband, boyfriend, baby daddy—he should see it all. Let him stomach the view. That's the price they pay since they get the easy end of this pregnancy bit. Let them see what your body ultimately goes through to bear their offspring.

With that rant out of the way, this is probably a really good time to refresh your memory on all the behind-the-scenes perks of pregnancy. Rule number 1: You have the ultimate excuse for everything. "Enjoy the perks of pregnancy," says Angela from Washington, D.C. "If you don't milk it, even just a little bit, then you're really missing out." I've asked strangers for spare food in the name of pregnancy. Husbands and partners will do things they would never ordinarily do for you when you are pregnant. Revel in the temporary rebirth of chivalry. Enjoy being the focus of attention. Use those special parking spaces at the supermarket for expectant moms. Let people hold doors for you. Cut long bathroom lines. When eating, have seconds and thirds and nobody will look at you funny. Milk it, girl. That's what I did and scores of your sisterfriends, too. And we loved every minute of it.

I remember having these crazed nesting periods where I would be in Home Depot at 10:00 at night, buying new types of baby room paint, flooring, fixtures, and other nonsense on impulse. Of course, because I didn't measure a window or guesstimate floor space before I left the house on a madcap mission, I would end up returning and exchanging stuff all the time. So there I stood with my huge football-shaped belly, on the Returns & Exchanges line with a pair of blinds that were the wrong everything. The line was barely moving, my feet were starting to hurt, and of course, I had to pee. I was about to turn into psychowoman. When it was finally my turn, the orange-apron-clad lady told me to walk *all* the way to the farthest end of the store to get the correct size blind in order to complete my exchange. This probably would have made sense to a normal person. But my pregnancy brain prevented me from thinking of this beforehand—my bad. But there was no way I was walking all the way back there into the DYI Neverland to fetch another set of blinds. So I smiled nicely, rubbed my belly, and told the apron chick that if I had to walk that far after waiting that long at this stage in my pregnancy, I might have this baby right now in the Lumber Department. She quickly picked up her handy intercom and asked an associate from blinds to bring my desired size to the front desk. Ain't technology grand? With all that you're going through, never be afraid to get a little "customer service" of your own.

MOCHA MIX: WHAT THE SISTERS SAY . . . ABOUT THE PREGNANCY JOURNEY

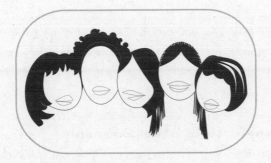

Pregnancy Fears

With your first child there is fear of the unknown. You've heard all the stories, but you still don't know what to expect. There's a fear of not knowing what YOU will feel like. But with that fear was a wonderful excitement that something is growing inside of me. —KUAE, MONTCLAIR, NEW JERSEY

People would ask if I was scared of giving birth. I was more scared of what to do after birth when I brought this baby home. The only thing that concerned me about birth was not knowing if I was really in labor. —LORRAINE, MABLETON, GEORGIA

What Surprised Me About Pregnancy

At first, I thought I would automatically be excited all the time. But preg–

nancy didn't feel the way I thought it would feel. It took about two months for me to settle in. —LYNETTE, LOUISVILLE, KENTUCKY

I didn't realize all that pregnancy involves. I never thought about the sleepless nights, and the work of calorie counting and healthy eating. There was so much planning. How will our financial situation be? What things can we be doing? It all took me by surprise. —IVY, SAINT LOUIS, MISSOURI

Finding Me-Time
I took prenatal aerobics and spent ten minutes reading every night. —SHAUN, OAKLAND, CALIFORNIA

I got weekly manicures and pedicures and a pregnancy massage once a month, or as needed. It was fabulous! —CYNTHIA, BROOKLYN, NEW YORK

The Strangest Thing About Pregnancy
Two things: a single, long hair grew from my nipple, and if I touched any raw meat, I absolutely couldn't eat it. My husband had to season, prepare, and cook any meats for us. —ESTHER, BALTIMORE, MARYLAND

My pelvis bone dislocated from the weight of the baby. It'd always been a troublesome area for me before pregnancy and as the pelvis loosened to prepare for labor, mine rotated a bit. I had to see a physical therapist twice a week, but that turned out to be a nice getaway. —JEANNE, SAINT LOUIS, MISSOURI

Best Pregnancy Advice
If you're lucky enough to get a day or two by yourself, go to the movies, sit in the bookstore, stroll the mall—you'll never have that leisure time in quite the same way ever again. —WENDY, LITTLE ROCK, ARKANSAS

My mother said to take the time and enjoy the pregnancy. We tend to always look forward to the next thing instead of enjoying where you are now. I was always reading about the next month instead of focusing on what was happening now. —LORRAINE, MABLETON, GEORGIA

Trust your body. You'll have a great pregnancy if you get out of your own way. And let your body do what it's doing. —ARIN, CHICAGO, ILLINOIS

ReTell Therapy

BUCK NAKED AND BEAUTIFUL

by Kuae Kelch Mattox

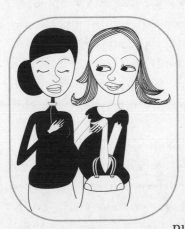

I've got a confession to make, and I must admit, I am smiling sheepishly as I think about it: When I was nine months pregnant, ten days before my son was born, I posed nude for a photographer. That's right; I stood in all my glory, belly protruding, breasts round and full, hair all done up, skin glistening with oil. Now, mind you, it wasn't for a steamy publication for mass male consumption. It was for a respected female photographer working on her own dream book project.

Even so, that was quite a leap for me, to step out of my otherwise ordinary life and do something that was, well, not so ordinary. It struck me especially, because, had anyone asked me to pose nude without being pregnant, I would have immediately scoffed at the idea. In fact, I would have rejected it outright.

So what brought about such a change in me? I guess I can only look to my roots. Growing up, my body image usually hovered between good and excellent. I always had what I considered to be a healthy body image. I was, quite simply, comfortable with my body. As a young girl, I remember being very skinny and sometimes a little awkward. But I credit my inspiring parents, and especially my mother, for teaching me that beauty is in the eye of the beholder, and that it comes in many forms. Of course, like many parents, they told me that I was beautiful on the outside, but they always made it a point to show me that the greatest beauty comes from within. My mother, the drama teacher, playwright, and romantic, would often share with fondness her own pregnancy stories, and my father, the professor and poet, would tell my brother, sister, and I that our entry into this world was the greatest gift that could ever have been bestowed upon him.

Together, their words and actions, always loving and supportive, were my role models, planting the seeds of confidence in my young, impressionable mind. As I got older and started to fill out, I remember as a teenager thinking my body was kind of cute and shapely. I didn't mind revealing a little, but I was never one to flaunt it, or even show it off. I always wanted to be dignified, elegant, and classy.

So that's why I was not prepared for this sudden change in mentality with pregnancy. What was it about pregnancy that had me gushing so much I now wanted to show off my body? I had heard the stories that so many women are eager to tell—Girl, you're not going to feel as sexy as you did before . . . wait till those stretch marks come . . . your ankles are going to be as big as a cow's . . . your skin is going to change . . . your butt is going to get big . . . if you lose your beauty, that means you're going to have a girl . . . in the end you're going to be begging that doctor to take that baby out.

Yet, as a pregnant woman (and I can say this with great certainty because I now have three children and I felt this with all three), not only did I feel physically beautiful, I literally glowed from within. It was as if someone, or something, was constantly shining a warm and glorious light around me. I seized every opportunity to marvel at myself in the mirror. I was one of those women who liked to touch her belly and rub it, savoring each and every movement that I felt inside. I carried myself with such an air of confidence. I even stood taller.

Then there was the emotional and spiritual icing, the knowledge that a most precious gift had been bestowed upon me. I felt, quite literally, that my body and my mind now had a higher calling. My self-image catapulted to a level that words could barely explain.

So one day in 1999, while I was working as a producer for NBC News, a fellow producer told me about a female photographer friend of hers who was working on a book about nude pregnant women. She said her friend had taken many pictures of nude pregnant women already but wanted more women of color. She thought I looked great and that I'd be a perfect subject for her friend.

I was very flattered at the suggestion, but the journalist in me was skeptical. Who was this photographer? Why is she taking pictures of nude pregnant women? What on earth could those pictures look like? Were they sleazy? Were they trashy? What's the point? I had a million questions when the photographer and I spoke.

She was patient and very detailed in her descriptions and explanations. It turned out she had always wanted to publish a book of photographs of nude, pregnant women in unusual locations, and she wanted the women to write down their feelings about being pregnant. A few days later, samples of her work were in my mailbox. I was completely blown away. The pictures, in black and white, were stunning—women of all shapes and sizes, some posing with delight, others with solemnity, in locations that I could not believe. There was a woman standing amidst a cornfield, a woman stretched over the top of her grand piano . . . a woman standing in the middle of the Brooklyn Bridge. The pictures had been taken at different times of the day, so the natural light gave the images an undeniably organic quality and the shadows and shadings made each picture look like a true work of art.

The next day's topic of conversation over dinner with my husband went something like this: "So honey, a friend of mine at work told me about a photographer who is working on a book about pregnant nude women and she'd like to shoot some pictures of me. What do you think?" Of course, the fork went down and the brow went up, but after sharing with him all that the photographer had shared with me, he felt comfortable, and he said the decision was really up to me.

It was almost a month before I called her back. Should I or shouldn't I? Ultimately, I knew that years from now I would be angry with myself if I didn't. And although she could never fully capture the beauty that I felt, I knew that a picture of me in all my pregnant glory would always evoke a sweet memory that would linger for the rest of my life. Just like a smell years later—my dad's pipe tobacco, for instance—can evoke memories of childhood, so, too, could a picture, a visual image, conjure up the powerful way that I felt during pregnancy.

After scouting several locations with meticulous details in mind, we selected an old train station with a historic ticket house near my home. Hundreds, maybe thousands, of residents, pass through that station every day on their way to work in New York City. The plan was for me to pose early in the morning standing on the train tracks . . . I was ready.

It was a blistering cold November day when I woke at the crack of dawn. It was such a strange feeling to shower, smooth moisturizer over my body, and then cover myself with only a winter coat. My heart was not pounding. I was not nervous. I was so calm, and so sure that this was what I wanted to do.

As I stood on those tracks and removed my coat, I remember a rush of cold air swept over my body. There were those few moments of self-consciousness when I wondered if any early morning commuters were watching. Then came a few deep breaths, and as the shutter clicked away, a sheer feeling of liberation.

What she captured in her lens, and what ultimately became the photo that we selected, still brings tears to my eyes. It is a portrait of calm, beauty, and grace that I will never forget. Every once in a while, I take a look at my picture. When I look at it, I am that pregnant woman again, full of optimism and hope for my children, feeling whole, at peace with my life and myself. One day, I will show my picture to my children, with the hope that they, too, will feel the beauty that I felt as they grew inside of me. Just as my mother taught me about the beauty that is pregnancy, I hope the picture speaks volumes to my children as well.

GOT NEWS?
When and How to Make the Big Announcement

*Y*ou've got big news and you want to shout it from the mountaintops. But should you? The general rule of thumb has always been to wait until after the first trimester, when the risk of miscarriage drops drastically. Some people only want to tell their immediate family before that time for fear of an early pregnancy loss. Others tell everyone, reasoning that if they did have a loss, they would want the support of others. Choosing the whens and hows of making your announcement can feel tricky. Here are a few tips:

Your Family: Try as you might to wait, family members have a way of figuring these things out pretty quickly. You may even give yourself away if you have severe nausea and vomiting. Or there's always an intuitive auntie or grandmother who comments on your "smell" of pregnancy, or something equally odd that tells her you are with child.

It was Big Mama who told Diane, from Long Beach, California, that she was pregnant long before she even knew. Big Mama said you could always tell that a black woman is pregnant by the double pulse in her neck, and Diane's neck had it. Diane blew it off as an old wives' tale (read more on these in Chapter Three), but when her period didn't come the following week, she was too curious to wait. A pregnancy test proved her Big Mama right. So, don't be surprised when well-intentioned country folk call you out.

If family members keep asking before you're ready to share and you don't want to lie, try saying, "Well, we're definitely putting in the practice," or "I wouldn't mind if I were," or "No announcements to be made." Just remember: don't feel pressured. Share the news when you and your partner feel comfortable. Here's an idea: call your mom and tell her to set another place at Thanksgiving dinner next year.

Your Friends: Sharing with your closest friends can be your best revelations. Hugs, kisses, gifts, and free lunches are sure to come your way. If not, get new friends! When sharing, start off with the friend you are absolutely, 100 percent sure will be over the moon for you. If you're not elated yet about this pregnancy, then tell the friend who's always able to look at things positively. For a fun group announcement with friends, invite them over for a cocktail party and drink milk from your martini glass. They'll be sure to figure it out.

Your Job: Most women advise holding off telling your job for as long as possible. That gives you time to do some research and preparation and decreases the months you feel your work performance is under a microscope. Before you tell your boss:

1. Research your employer's health plan and parental leave policy. Check out the company Web site, anonymously call human resources or the personnel department, or check with your union rep. Get the specifics on what type of paid and unpaid leave you may be eligible for. Some companies offer some unpaid leave that still includes benefits. And tell your man to get cracking, too—dads are now eligible for family leave.

2. Allow your pregnancy to progress. Two or three months can give your doctor some indication as to whether complications or special needs are likely to develop. These factors can affect the time off you may need before and after the birth.

3. Don't automatically assume you'll just take the standard leave and that's it. It may be hard to imagine what life will be like with a new baby. Sure, your career-minded self says, I need to be back at the office, but the new mommy self may want as much time as possible at home. And if that's financially possible—a very real option after reading the financial guide in Chapter Twelve—then why not? As you prepare to discuss your pregnancy and leave, include several different scenarios. That gives your boss a framework for creating a flexible plan. For example, come up with three-month, six-month, and twelve-month leave options. Even if it doesn't happen, think it

through. Better to have an idea of how it can work earlier on than to wait until your hands are full with a new baby.

4. Pick a good time to talk to your boss. Ask her assistant what other activities, deadlines, or travel commitments are coming up so you can pick a day when he's not rushing, stressed out, or in a plain ole bad mood. Depending on your relationship with your boss and the company policy, you may write her a letter instead. Either way, be sure to express your commitment and long-term interest in your job and the company. Employers can be more generous when they don't sense that you're about to jump ship.

Your Partner

These days, most men know their woman's cycle like their own. Just when you are about to forget your period is coming, your partner will remind you. My friend Rashaun's fiancé routinely pops a maxipad into her purse for her on the appropriate day. So when many of us are late and then inevitably pregnant, there's not much surprise left because he asks every day, "Did it come yet?" or calls the job, "Did it come yet?" Ten minutes later, "What about now?" It's worse than that "Can you hear me now?" commercial. And with home pregnancy tests, your partner is more likely to be around when you find out. If you've managed to keep the news to yourself, try leaving the pregnancy test out where he'll find it; better yet, gift wrap it. Or send him a Father's Day card and say congratulations. Even if it doesn't feel like fresh news, that doesn't mean you still can't try something unique once you have confirmation. Here are some techniques other sisters used:

My husband was working late so I just left the pregnancy test on the sink in the bathroom. When he came home and saw it, he was so excited. He started jumping up and down on the bed. He was like a kid at Christmas. —Phyllis, Chicago, Illinois

We had a number of false alarms in the past. So when the test was positive, my husband looked me in the eye, with a serious face, and said, "Take it again." He got me another test, and it was positive. Then he felt okay to get excited. —TIA, SAINT LOUIS, MISSOURI

My husband made the biggest boo-boo. He got so excited he couldn't wait until we left the doctor's office to tell his family. Since his cell phone couldn't get enough reception to make a call, he quickly and foolishly sent off a round of text messages. He thought he was giving them real-time information. I thought it was a stupid idea. His family felt offended that he shared such big news with an impersonal text message. I was upset that he ruined our big moment with his impetuousness. —LISA, LITHONIA, GEORGIA

I told one of my girlfriends and swore her to secrecy. She didn't tell, but when I told the rest of our friends, instead of acting surprised, she blurted that she "been knew." My other friends felt slighted and hurt. If you have a sister crew, tell them all pretty much at the same time. —JANEEN, CHARLESTON, SOUTH CAROLINA

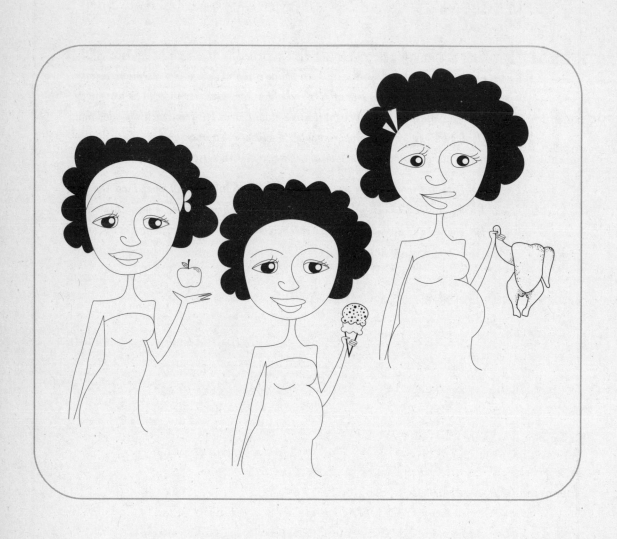

2

The Pregnancy Lowdown

A Trimester-by-Trimester Guide

Are you ready? Your body is ready to fulfill its biological imperative and you're just along for the ride. And ten months—that's right, forty weeks is really ten months—is a long time. But with so much going on and so much to do, it will, amazingly, pass very quickly. One day soon, the journey of pregnancy will just be a fond memory to share with others, but in the meantime there will be a lot going on.

Just as each trimester is different in the ways your baby grows and develops, each trimester introduces different changes to your emotions, your body, and your ability to manage your job—whether that's as a mom or a manager.

So with the help of some girlfriends, some experts, and some common sense I've put together a road map of what to expect when you don't know what the hell to expect for the next ten months.

We'll look at each trimester, with a focus on your mind—your emotions and worries and what to do about them; your body—how your body is changing and expanding and how to adjust and get comfortable with this new you; your baby—how little junior is developing and growing; and your job—tips on juggling work and pregnancy, and preparing for maternity leave. Let's get started.

First Trimester
(Conception to Fourteen Weeks)

Your Mind

You're probably feeling really emotional these days. Things that didn't bother you before may cause you to dissolve into tears. Some women report an intense crankiness, disgust with their husband or partner, and a general feeling they were "losing it." In fact, you're probably having all the signs of PMS—the bloating, mood swings, cramping, backaches—without the eventual arrival of your period. By the time your second and third months roll by, you'll be ripe with feelings of anxiety, fear, excitement, depression, guilt, and happiness—all in the space of about seven minutes. You are beginning to experience the emotional roller-coaster ride of pregnancy. For most of us it starts with the scary realization that life is about to be changed permanently; this may make you happy or this may make you sad, or, thanks to the pregnancy hormones, you may be both at the same time.

Your Body

Even though there aren't any visible signs of pregnancy yet, your body has undergone a lot of changes already—the uterus has formed a lush bed of tissue; within hours of Mr. Sperm's meeting Ms. Egg, your baby's gender, eye color, and hair texture have been set; and your little fertilized egg has traveled all the way through the fallopian tube and into the uterus—it's no wonder you're feeling more tired. Once that egg has reached its final resting spot in the uterus, it triggers the production of human chorionic gonado-tropin (hCG), the hormone that turns your pregnancy test result positive and your life upside down. Pumped-up levels of estrogen and progesterone are also being produced. All of this happens before week four, when you miss your period or have some slight spotting.

Your body may be giving you other signs as well, swelling, queasiness, and frequent trips to the bathroom. Many black women, including me, have a mole outbreak.

A big clue for Joyce, from Houston, Texas, was a ravenous appetite. "I was hungry every three hours on the dot. I would wake up in the middle of the night hungry and need a snack. I would clear my dinner plate and start eyeballing my husband's food." If you find yourself hungry enough to gnaw on your own flesh, by all means eat. But go for something healthy instead of heading for the tub of ice cream.

You may also notice that you feel short of breath or that you need to take more deep breaths to feel comfortable. That's because the amount of air you inhale in each breath decreases by 40 percent when you're pregnant, so you need to breathe in more air to get enough oxygen to you and your baby. Doctors aren't sure why this happens, but they think it may be set off by that pesky proges-terone hormone that's invading your body. Don't worry that you're not getting enough oxygen: your body knows exactly what it's doing.

Around the tenth week, parts of your eye become thicker and swollen with fluid (I told you pregnancy affects everything!). Your vision won't change, but you may have problems wearing contacts or they just won't feel comfortable. For the time being, wear glasses. Typically, your eyes will resume their original shape about six weeks after delivery.

These minor changes may make you anxious about the more dramatic body changes ahead. This is a good time to talk about exercising during pregnancy. Any exercise program should be approved by your doctor. And any doctor worth his copay will tell you never to take up a new or more difficult regimen than you've been regularly doing. In the early days of pregnancy, things are still pretty delicate, and exercise can be risky. Weigh your options and the risks. Second of all—and this is my biggie—you're going to get fat anyway. Pregnancy should be about indulging yourself, letting go (within reason), and not trying to control everything. To me, it seems most of the pregnant women who are on the treadmills and lifting miniweights need group therapy for control freaks.

There's also a strange belief lurking about that exercise helps you have an easier delivery. Well, I've spoken to hundreds of your sisthren and not one of them said she was better prepared for all the pushing, grunting, and bearing down involved with delivery because of doing lunges and lifting one-pound weights. Sara, from Rochester, New York, however, is convinced that exercise helped her stamina during labor. "I definitely feel like exercising during pregnancy helped me last longer during labor. I didn't tire so quickly. I felt limber. And if nothing else, it helped my mind game because I felt more confident about my body strength." There are plenty of women whose only form of exercise was lifting heaping spoons of ice cream into their mouth, yet they walked into the hospital, pushed out a baby in three grunts, and were on their merry way. I share this to remind you that there are no hard-and-fast rules or guarantees when it comes to this pregnancy business.

Your Baby
Your baby goes from superstar swimming sperm, to a *zygote*—the term used to describe a fertilized egg in the first four days—to an *embryo*, the term for your baby until about ten weeks' gestation. By the second month, its poppy-seed-size heart is beating, other major organs are forming, and your uterus is growing to about the size of a peach. Your baby is looking more like a tadpole than a human. It's flat and it has a tail and only limb buds.

Your tiny embryo graduates to full fetus status by month three, and you'll be introduced to one of the new rituals of pregnancy: cold goo. It seems that all baby exams require supercold goo slathered on your belly, and few people try to warm it up. Your first experience with the cold goo will probably be while hearing the baby's heartbeat by using a sound-wave stethoscope called a Doppler. The cold goo will also be used for future sonograms. I like to call it the Shock and Aaaahhh!! Maneuver. First they shock you with the subzero goo, and then as soon as you hear that baby's heartbeat or see the image of a sonogram you forget about the shock and melt into a sappy "Aaaahhh" over the sound or sight of your precious baby. It works everytime. Hearing your baby's heartbeat for the very first time will likely be one of the most thrilling "firsts" of your pregnancy—I took a tape recorder along the first time. Don't be frightened by how fast a baby's heartbeat is, about one hundred forty to one hundred sixty times per minute—are they running a marathon in there?—as this is normal and expected.

By the ninth week or so, the brain is growing like gangbusters. The head makes up half of the fetus's total length from the top of the head to the butt. The baby looks more like E.T. than a cute, cuddly baby, but it's still early days. By the end of the third month, your baby will double in length, have separate fingers instead of ones that are webbed, have all facial features including eyelids that have opened and then fused shut by a thin membrane, have arms, legs, thighs, and teeny toes. Meanwhile, your baby is taking his first stab at doing something that'll probably gross you out—drinking his own urine. The baby is now producing urine that is released into the amniotic fluid. Some of that fluid is reabsorbed and the fetus swallows it, but it is sterile and harmless.

Your Job

Just as pregnancy changes a lot of personal relationships, it can give your work life a real overhaul as well. With all the sick days caused by morning sickness, time away for medical appointments, workplace stress, and the like, managing pregnancy and work at the same time is a challenge. Studies show that certain activities and working conditions can increase your risk of having preterm labor or giving birth to a low-birth-weight baby. If your job requires heavy, repetitive lifting; prolonged standing; long and stressful commutes; or exposure to heavy vibrations, such as from large machines, you may need to talk to your doctor about special precautions. You should also be concerned if you're a schoolteacher, child-care worker, health care professional, or veterinary worker since these jobs can expose you to infections from adults, animals, or the worst germ carriers known to Earth—small children. Exposure to chicken pox and German measles, also known as rubella, can be dangerous for a pregnant woman. Talk to your doctor about some infection-control measures.

You're probably pulling your hair out trying to figure out how to get to your doctor and back on your lunch hour. Or you have a test or a sonogram and you've been sitting there waiting for thirty minutes for your technician, getting really nervous because you hope nobody at the office notices that you've been gone for two hours already. It's stressful. Did you know that in Ireland, your employer is required to let you off and pay you for time to take parenting classes and however much time you need for prenatal visits? Yep, no sneaking around. No eating your lunch under your desk because you spent your lunchtime at a doctor appointment. No checking voicemail while you're waiting in that white gown for the doctor to enter the exam room. Must be nice.

One of the best tools in managing your workplace while pregnant is actually knowing and understanding your workplace. Every office has a culture, a personality, a vibe that permeates the place. What is the nature of your work beast? Is it supportive and mom-friendly, or do you have a Nazi-like boss? Do you work with a bunch of culturally insensitive old frat boys (who may at least have a wife and kids at home) or some equally insensitive young frat guys (who find pregnancy, in their vernacular, "gross!")? Are there any other mothers on staff, or have they all quit in frustration? I've found that in some male-dominated workplaces, they may pay a lot of lip service to supporting pregnancy and being family friendly, but they expect you to be at your business-as-usual best. In some of these frat boy places, when a guy takes a day off for a hangover, it's totally acceptable, but taking a day off for morning sickness is a career limiting move. And what about workplace risks? Do you work around smokers who defy all the federal laws (you know the ones that are posted on all the walls) about not smoking in the workplace? Are you usually expected to lift heavy boxes of paper, office supplies, files, and other stuff? What if you're one of those three bags a day women I see on the train commuting to work? They have an overloaded briefcase brimming with papers, a stuffed large tote bag on the shoulder, *and* a purse. What is up with that? I've always wanted to jump on these women, pimp slap them with a *Real Simple* magazine, and shout, THAT'S JUST TOO MUCH STUFF!!!! But I digress. The point is, carrying heavy boxes, briefcases, and bags is even crazier if you're pregnant. It can put your baby at risk and you'll already have enough to carry around.

Travel can be another problem. If you're plagued with terrible morning sickness and nausea, it's kind of hard to do your usual O. J. Simpson sprint through the airport. Do you know how many gag-inducing smells you'll pass on the way to gate 11? Not to mention, the energy it takes to pack and the thought of being ten thousand feet above ground trapped in a germ-infested vessel with no fresh air for hours. God forbid you should hit turbulence and have to endure twenty minutes of rocky shaking—the last thing you need with a delicate stomach. My girlfriend Schalawn, who put in thirteen years as a flight attendant, gave me two tips when I was pregnant: sit in the middle of the plane, never the back, for a smoother ride, and never drink the water or any tea or coffee on board. As she put it, the water quality on airplanes is "suspect."

I had a big problem with flight anxiety in my first trimester—and I'm the kind of person who would hop a transatlantic flight with no problem. Just the thought of going up into the air made me anxious and literally sick. Of course, I couldn't explain this to my editor when he insisted I travel from New York City to L.A. to do an interview for my next story. I couldn't even rely on my usual flight anxiety reducer—a Jack Daniels and Coke—to help me. After a number of excuses and delays, I had to go. I prayed to make it through, but I was still crying during takeoff and restless for the entire flight. The whole thing was so stressful for me. Luckily, that phase passed.

Talk to your doctor about your traveling demands, especially if you have a medical condition, or have a history of miscarriages, or are considered high risk for any other reason. When traveling by plane or by car, take breaks to move around frequently. Get up and take a walk. This can help minimize any risk of swelling in the legs and blood clots. Try flexing and stretching your calves while seated. Either way, remember that most airlines won't allow you on board if you're past your thirty-sixth week, and most foreign airlines will show you the door at thirty-five weeks. Of course, being typical brown superwomen, a lot of sisters report flying beyond those dates by wearing a long, camouflaging trench coat or carrying one in front of their stomach.

Back at the office, you may also be anxious about being "mommy tracked." A lot of us black women have a need to accomplish things, and our work-related achievements may play a big role in our self-identity. Perhaps our five-year plan for taking over the corporate offices, renaming the company after ourselves, and giving all the black folks a secret raise didn't really factor in a pregnancy. We may view our pregnancy as just a temporary side stop in our continued upward climb to senior management, but senior management may see motherhood as a lifetime liability. I met a marketing executive from Chicago who was fired from her high-profile job a few weeks before her due date. That's definitely shady. A number of women had just started a new job and were obsessed with "proving" themselves to their employer. They dreaded telling their bosses and thinking about how they were perceived in terms of future promotions and assignments. Whether you've been at the job for ten days or ten years, the sad truth is that most black people don't have the kind of unspoken job security that comes when your daddy's old college buddy is in upper management. These are all the things that can bring on anxiety in the early days.

Sheryl, an urban marketing executive at a record label, was used to dealing with high-maintenance artists and crunked-out rappers. But her biggest challenge occurred when she became pregnant after a year on the job. "There were only two women in the company with children, and the general manager who set up the maternity policies was single, no children, and didn't have a clue," she says. "There were no work from home policies, no extended leave options. It was a battle." "Men don't have to deal with this career versus family struggle," says Vanessa, an attorney from Washington, D.C. "No one ever questions if a man will 'check out' just because he had a child." It's enough to make you want to holler.

Just when I was stressed out with all the tumbling thoughts about managing work and the future, I learned an important lesson at my four-year-old daughter's Winter Concert. I was pregnant at the time, so therefore I was crying. This time, out of sentimentality about my daughter, growing up, moving on, and singing her heart out up there on stage. Well, it vaguely resembled singing. But it was about eight four-year-olds doing their tone-deaf best. Once I blocked out the sounds that mimic those that only dogs can hear, and the kids who were just saying Blah, Blah, Blah to the beat, I finally heard the words to "Whistle While You Work." They were quite simple. "When there's too much to do, don't let them bother you. Just do your best and take a rest and sing yourself a song." Who knew the greatest career guidance for my pregnancy would come from Seven Dwarfs? Any time thereafter when I felt myself getting overwhelmed about work, I would sing a relaxing tune, or better yet, call my daughter and ask her to sing that one for me. This became particularly challenging at the office, where every time I tried to hum something tranquil my mind drifted to the black folks' official workplace anthem—"Y'all gonna make me lose my mind, up in here, up in here." But you really can't over-worry about your career or being slighted at the office. It doesn't do you or your baby any good. In the meantime, try these more practical tips for office survival:

* Think like you're on the airplane: Know your exits and the nearest bathroom. You never know when a spontaneous crying fit or vomiting spree may hit. Being able to identify the nearest stairwell, supply closet, or vacant cubicle or office when the tears swell, and the nearest bathroom when you start gagging, will be helpful.

* Adjust your routine. As you now know, morning sickness can last all day. And it's hard to attend a meeting, write a report, or train staff when you're barfing your insides out. It's even worse when you're not barfing, but have that barf reflex, with the sound, and the body spasms, but nothing coming out—not exactly your power presentation for the office. You may feel stressed because you haven't told your boss, yet your sickness is affecting work. The first thing is to remember you can't pop out of bed, run through the shower, and get to work anymore. In fact, rushing around in the morning can make you even queasier. You need more time to manage the morning sickness. Try waking up a little earlier to get your morning sickness rebuff routine down pat. If you find that eating two saltines followed by a green Now 'N' Later and a shot of ginger ale works for you, give yourself time to do it. If possible, try to relax your morning work routine. Do you hold 7:30 A.M. staff meetings? (God, I hope you're not that cruel.) You might need to switch them to a later time. If you find yourself exhausted by the afternoon, get your toughest or high-concentration tasks out of the way in the morning.

* Start identifying an ally. This may be a good time to seek out an ally at the workplace—not the office gossip, but perhaps someone you can trust. I mean really trust. This is important because this can absolutely backfire if word of your pregnancy gets out. The last thing you want is for your boss to find out about your pregnancy through the grapevine. "My assistant saved my ass," says Katrice, a public relations executive from New York City. "She covered my phone calls, made adjustments in my schedule

if I looked overtired, and always had a good answer for why I stepped away from my office."

✳ Delegate and accept help. This is a good time to start asking others for help. You don't have to do it all. And if someone offers to answer your phone while you close your door to grab a power nap, accept.

✳ Find a place for a nap, whether it's your office, the company medical room, your car, or at home. Denise Fleming, from Manassus, Virginia, had a girlfriend who lived near her office. She would just pop by for her midday naps. At some point, every pregnant girl needs a nap, even it's for twenty minutes.

✳ Be gracious and offer trade-offs. Some of your coworkers may feel that they are doing more than their fair share to cover for you, now that you're tired, off ill, or missing work because of doctor appointments. Try to make amends by being extra thankful of their extra work and offering to help them out when you're rested and have your energy back.

✳ Lighten up. Don't make an unrealistic schedule. Are you an active member of every professional, alumnae, religious, and civic group known to humankind? Do you sit on the board of a nonprofit organization? You may have to cut back on your extracurricular involvement to carve out time for rest and de-stressing.

✳ Dig out your sense of humor. It may be the only thing that saves you sometimes. And whatever happens, know that despite your best efforts to be professional, there's still a strong chance one of your colleagues will inevitably walk into your office and find you facedown, asleep on your desk, drooling all over your desk calendar.

Second Trimester
(Fourteen to Twenty-eight Weeks)

Your Mind

Around this time, women notice the onslaught of pregnancy brain. You can't complete your sentences. You've locked your keys, yourself, or your purse in the car on three separate occasions in one week. Or worse, people tell you something, walk away, and you can't recall the faintest notion of what they just said to you. Don't worry; thousands of pregnant women have been there. In fact, I will say that my brain has yet to resume its full thinking and memory capacity. Three words of advice: Post-it notes. From here on in, you have to write everything down. Do not trust your memory anymore. It is not the faithful companion it once was. Get a diary, a pocket notepad, a cocktail napkin (since you won't need it for a cocktail!). I also had to establish a triple-check routine every time I left the house—purse, keys, cell phone. No matter how much I tried, inevitably once a week I would end up on the commuter train without my monthly pass, in my office lobby with no work ID, or at the register with lunch in hand only to realize I'd forgotten my money.

By this time, now that the riskiest period for miscarriage has passed, you're probably itching to tell everyone on the street your good news. Also, your own anxiety about a possible miscarriage may lessen now. With luck your nausea and vomiting are subsiding and you may feel renewed, ready to do things and resume some outside activities. You may be feeling downright sexy! But resist the temptation to overdo it, now that you've got your stride back.

I've found that increased vulnerability strikes during this period, and you feel more emotionally dependent on your partner. Maybe it has something to do with the pregnancy's being more obvious, and the increased weight gain; I'm not sure, but a lot of women also said they needed more attention and reassurance from their man, and from friends and relatives. Around this time, every woman has some sort of issue about the weight gain. If you were skinny, you may be excited by your rounder body or depressed by it. If you're overweight or have been battling your weight, you may be less excited and may be anxious about being even bigger than you already are. With all of these feelings afloat, this is not the time to ask your partner, "Honey, do I look fat?" No answer will satisfy you.

Your Body

Say bye-bye to your waistline; it's disappearing by now and won't be back any time soon. From here on out, you'll be gaining about a half pound to a pound every week; at least so say those charts I've grown to despise. You may be outgrowing the safety-pinned and rubber-banded waistbands and be about ready to break out the maternity clothes—but don't go before reading Chapter Nine on pregnancy style! If the extra fat deposits weren't enough, your rib cage is enlarging to make space for your increasing lung capacity. By the time you deliver, the distance around your rib cage will have expanded by two to three inches.

The good news is that at about twenty weeks, a sonogram can detect the baby's gender, that is, if the little bugger plays nice and doesn't have its legs folded up. For many, finding out what they are having finally makes the whole thing real—as if vomiting, weight gain, and devouring every snack that isn't bolted down weren't enough.

Your breasts are still ballooning; this will continue until the fifth month. Your nipples are getting bigger, and pimplelike bumps may appear. Believe it or not, they have a name: glands of Montgomery. These are oil-producing glands that help protect the skin on the nipples from drying out and cracking.

This is also the trimester when lots of women report bleeding gums, since more blood circulates there, making them soft, swollen, and spongy. Simple brushing and flossing may spark bleeding, but continue to brush twice a day using a soft toothbrush.

Carlise, a teacher from Trenton, New Jersey, had sharp pains in her lower abdomen during her second trimester. "It totally freaked me out, and it turned out I had round ligament pain. I had no clue about round ligaments before," she says. Round ligaments are attached from the pelvis to each side of the uterus. As your uterus grows, they become stretched, and, as you'll be learning through this pregnancy, stretching can equal hurting. Note: moving from side to side or trying to roll over suddenly while sleeping can make it worse. Try to avoid any sudden movements and take a warm bath or use a hot water bottle on the area. Doctors recommend sleeping in the fetal position, with a pillow underneath your belly and between your knees to support your top leg.

There's also more activity in dem bones, as the ligaments supporting your abdomen continue to stretch and the joints between your pelvic bones soften and loosen up in anticipation of childbirth. Your lower spine gets into the mix by continuing to curve backward (you know the infamous pregnancy stance) to prevent you from falling forward from the weight of your cargo. All those loose joints combined with a changed center of gravity, and less experience dealing with this new expanded body, make for increased clumsiness.

Headaches can make a special appearance this trimester, thanks to the high levels of hormones in effect. Stress, dehydration, lack of sleep, eyestrain, and hunger can also cause headaches. Don't reach for your favorite pain reliever; remember, most aren't allowed. Try a light snack, some water, and a power nap in a dark room. Think about reducing stress or try to take a fifteen-minute break every few hours or so at work or at home to sit quietly and do some deep breathing exercises. Make sure you're getting enough sleep at night. If the headaches persist, call your doctor.

You may get your sexual desire back, too, now that you're getting used to this new pregnancy body. With your new curves and girth, sex can be awkward and clumsy, but don't let that put you off. Keep trying.

Your Baby

Your fetus begins this trimester looking like a fully formed tiny human, with an out-of-proportion E.T.-sized head, and by the sixth month your baby will be gaining weight rapidly, kicking, and tumbling. Most women reported feeling their first wallop in their belly between twenty and twenty-three weeks. The sensation of your baby's first movements is commonly called "quickening." You may also notice your baby's thrusts, stretching, and side-to-side tosses and arm movements though you may not know what that feeling is the first time it happens. But by the end of the fifth month the baby is up to a pound in weight and about twelve inches long by the end of the month, and he's ready to make his presence known. He has already been practicing breathing and may even be sucking his thumb. He can hear now, so it may be time to swap your hip hop compilation for a little Mozart in the CD changer. There are loads of studies on the connection between Mozart's music and its good effects on a baby's brain development. Some studies have linked listening to Mozart to improved math skills. It could be a whole lot of hooey, but I'm a believer and could be readily found in my office with headphones around my belly and some Mozart in the CD player.

By about week twenty, the placenta, which delivers food and oxygen to your baby and takes away waste, is fully formed. And by the end of the fifth month, your little girl will have a uterus, ovaries, and a vagina that begins to open. Your little boy's testes begin to lower from the abdomen into the scrotum.

During the sixth month, your baby really starts to look like a, well, baby—or at least a wrinkled version thereof. That giant head isn't so big in proportion to the rest of her body, hair on the head and eyebrows begins to grow, fingernails appear, the lungs are developing rapidly, taste buds appear, and your baby's brain and nerve endings are now developed enough to understand the sensation of a touch. By now, those fluttering feelings of movement have graduated to full-out Tae Bo kicks.

Your Job

As I've mentioned, in all the conversations I've had with women, from corner office executives to shift workers at the local manufacturing companies, the one thing almost 100 percent advised was to keep your pregnancy a secret for as long as possible. Lisa, a Wall Street trader, told her boss in January, and she was due in March. Her trick? "Sweaters. Lots of sweaters." Depending on your job, and the season, you may be able to hold off. If you haven't told the boss, then you're probably living a strange double life. Hiding your pregnancy by day, and then taking time to enjoy, relish, and explore your changing body when you get home. When I returned from a secret sonogram appointment wearing a Kool-Aid smile, coworkers would ask why I was so happy. It was hard to put on my game face when my bag contained an image of my precious cargo.

Being pregnant in the winter lets you cover up with cozy turtlenecks, thick sweaters, pashmina shawls, and lots of blazers. This isn't so easy if it's summertime. One of my tricks was to invite people to my office, where I could hide behind my desk, instead of going to their office. If I had to go to another person's office for a meeting, I would immediately sit down.

Another issue is socializing. For more and more women, entertaining clients or socializing with colleagues is an important part of the job. So what do you do when your male boss wants you to take a client out for drinks and you can't drink? Or worse, you are out with your boss and the rest of the sales team celebrating some new deal and you won't have your usual martini toast? Suzanne, from Los Angeles, would conveniently make a long trip to the ladies' room and then feign disgust that she had missed the toast when she returned. Chantal from Detroit just avoided those occasions altogether, making out that she had previous plans that could not be changed. But she admits that strategy backfired because not hanging out with the boys cost her new projects. Anyone who works in that type of environment knows that most work assignments are made at the bar or on the golf course. One strategy that worked for me was to think like a frat boy. What do most of them relate to? Drinking—excessively. So when hanging out with the guys at work and offered a drink I would say, "Oh no, I can't. Last night, I went out for drinks with some people from _____ (marketing, sales, company XYZ), and we got so wasted, if I have one more sip I'll have to go directly to Betty Ford. I'm on a serious detox." Everyone understands a hangover. On another occasion, a colleague bought me a drink, which I graciously accepted and held in my hand. I never drank it but used it as a prop as I made my socializing rounds and then I just put it down somewhere before I took my leave.

Stay clever. A rum and Coke looks the same as a Diet Coke in a glass. And a cranberry juice with a shot of club soda looks just like a vodka cranberry in your hand—especially if you tell people that's what it is!

Keep in mind: maternity leave is closer than you think. If you haven't already done so, start now to build and strengthen the relationships that will be crucial for a successful maternity leave. Practice give-and-take among coworkers, with more giving on your part as you try to build up a reservoir of goodwill that you can tap in your final trimester when things get tough and while you are out on maternity leave. While you're having a boost of energy this trimester, do what you can reasonably do to demonstrate your vital contribution to the department.

As you progress this trimester, everyday things like sitting, bending, standing, and lifting become a bit more uncomfortable. Your growing bundle of joy is feeling more like a ball of pain as it causes constant pressure on your bladder, a strain on your back, and water retention in your legs and feet. If you have an office job, the chair you sit in is really important during pregnancy. The weight of your body is increasing and shifting, so a seat that can adjust for height and tilt is best. Adjustable armrests, back cushions, and good back support can make long hours of sitting more bearable. They also make life easier when you get to the point that getting out of a chair takes on the difficulty level of an Olympic sport.

* If you have a long driving commute, you may want to buy one of those lower-back support cushions.
* When sitting, elevate your feet on a footrest or box to take some of the strain off your back. This may also help reduce swelling in the feet and legs.
* Don't sit with your legs crossed.
* Don't stand for a long time. With all the increased dilatation of blood vessels during pregnancy, standing can cause blood to collect in the legs, and that can lead to pain, dizziness, and even fainting.
* If standing is part of your job, put one foot on a box or low stool to take pressure off your back and decrease blood pooling. If your job requires you to stand for four or more hours, be sure to talk to your doctor, who may want you to stop working earlier in your pregnancy.

If you've already announced your pregnancy to your boss, you may feel as if a load has been lifted off your shoulders. Carrying around a secret can be hard work for a woman! But you may also feel that people are treating you differently. "I noticed that three- and four-month projects were being handed off to less qualified people and I was only four months pregnant at the time. I had enough time to complete the task, but there was an 'oh-she's-risky-what-if-something-happens' factor involved," explains Kiana, who works in state education administration and lives in Burlington, New Jersey. Or you may feel that your superiors are less focused on your long-term training or career advancement. That's not your typical black folks paranoia acting up again. Recent studies in the United States and London showed that employers were not inclined to give pregnant workers additional training or grooming for higher positions—training they deemed useless since the woman was about to take leave and might not return afterward. There are two schools of thought here. You may feel flabbergasted that your boss assumed pregnancy rendered you any less a superwoman and spend the rest of your pregnancy stressing yourself out trying to prove him wrong. Or you can take it with a welcome sigh of relief. Your boss just actually did what you couldn't, but really should, do for yourself—lightened your workload. It may not be right, but it can work to your advantage. This is not necessarily the time to try to prove to the world that you can take on your full responsibilities to the bitter end, return to your desk exactly three months after giving birth, and pick up on the same rung where you left off climbing the corporate ladder.

But if you feel you are actually being discriminated against because of being pregnant or you were in line for a promotion prior to announcing your pregnancy and are now being told "We decided to go in another direction," you do have rights. The Pregnancy Discrimination Act of 1978 was passed as an amendment to the Civil Rights Act of 1964. In fact, thousands of women who are pregnant or new moms file charges every year with the Equal Employment Opportunity Commission. The law states that "women affected by pregnancy, childbirth, or related medical conditions shall be treated the same for all employment related purposes, including receipt of benefits under fringe benefit programs, as other persons not so affected but similar in their ability or inability to work." What that means without all the legalese is that your employer must treat you as well as he or she treats other workers who can't do their job for a short time because of, say, a broken leg or a heart attack. Just as that employee would be entitled to paid or unpaid disability leave (depending on company policy), you must also have this right if you are unable to work because of pregnancy or childbirth. And if pregnancy prevents you from being able to do your job, you have the right to be given easier duties. Employers are also not allowed to take away credit for previous years, accrued retirement benefits, vacation time, pay increases, or seniority because of a pregnancy-related disability.

Find out whether your state has a law about *temporary disability insurance* (at last check, California, Hawaii, New Jersey, New York,

Rhode Island, and Puerto Rico do), which offers partial wages during time off from work for medical problems, including those of pregnancy.

THE THIRD TRIMESTER
(TWENTY-EIGHT TO FORTY WEEKS)

Your Mind

You're almost there. This is the part they call the homestretch, and *stretch* will be the operative word here. Your belly will stretch beyond your imagination, as your baby makes its final growth spurt. At this point, you're probably enrolled in or about to start a childbirth class, which may have your mind lingering on the eternal question of all pregnant women: "Exactly how much will it hurt to get this person out of me? I mean, is it stump-your-toe pain or Brazilian bikini wax pain?" I was petrified of how much pain would be required to bring this baby into the world and many days I wished to stay pregnant forever. That's how scared I was. Pregnant women all over the world spend the final months trying to get some sort of varied sampling of painometer readings from every woman who has ever given birth. But the good thing about this birthing business in the new millennium is the most amazing and pivotal medical contribution to womankind—the epidural. That's right, ladies, I'm a pain punk and I like my epidural shaken not stirred and always on tap. "I would not go to the dentist and get a tooth pulled without a shot. Sure, back in the day, they just pulled teeth out of your head and operated on you while you were awake, but we don't do that anymore. And there's a good reason why we don't," says Denise from Manassus, Virginia. You too can rest easy knowing that this medical miracle is at your disposal. Now I know there are a lot of you out there who say you truly want to *experience* childbirth, the raw essence of it all in its gut wrenching glory. Well, a hearty hooty hooo, double soul clap, and a raise the roof for you. More power to ya, girl! But remember: there are no special stickers or door prizes for enduring hours of grueling pain. I like my deliveries the way God intended—heavily medicated from the waist down.

Whatever your labor plan is, it must be approved by your doctor. There may be aspects of your medical history—previous surgeries, high blood pressure, or uterine fibroids—that limit your labor options. For instance, if you have had a myomectomy or surgical removal of fibroids, your doctor may recommend a C-section. Some women can deliver vaginally after a myomectomy, but studies show that certain circumstances create a high risk for uterine rupture, which can lead to maternal death. A number of those circumstances relate to the depth and number of incisions made in the uterus and any postoperative infections, so if your current doctor did not do the surgical procedure, make sure he has full access to those records and to that surgeon if possible. Talk with both doctors and even get a third opinion if you still have doubts.

It's a good time to start preparing a list for your hospital bag. Your due date isn't set in stone and babies are notorious for showing up early. Pack as much as possible ahead of time, and keep a list of the last-minute items you'll need to throw in. And don't forget: you can't take a baby home without a car seat!

Your Body

Backaches, shortness of breath, and heartburn can really take over this trimester. The back pain may even spread down as far as the legs. That need to pee-pee all the time, which you noticed in the first trimester, will return with a vengeance, and you'll probably wear out the carpet between your bedroom and the bathroom before this is all over. Your stride will start to resemble the waddle that all pregnant women inevitably develop, and you may take two or three attempts to get out of a chair. Here are some other specifics:

The Uterus: By the beginning of the seventh month the uterus will reach roughly the midway point between your belly button and breasts. By the time this trimester ends, it will take up all the space from your pubic area to the bottom of your rib cage. Things start to liven up this trimester as the baby's kicks and punches increase, and practice contractions, called *Braxton-Hicks contractions*, start to occur. By the time this trimester ends your uterus will weigh twenty times more than its original two ounces and will have stretched to hold your baby, your placenta, and about a quart of amniotic fluid.

The Cervix: Somewhere around week thirty-seven, your cervix will begin to open or dilate. As this happens you may feel an occasional sharp, stabbing pain inside your vagina. A dilating cervix, at the right time, is good because that cervix needs to open from zero to ten centimeters in diameter before you can push the baby out.

Braxton-Hicks Contractions: This is the kind of stuff TV shows and movies are made of: A pregnant woman frantically wakes her husband, thinking she's in labor, and after her husband drives her to the hospital in his boxer shorts and with her suitcase on the roof, she's told it's just false contractions. Those pesky Braxton-Hicks have fooled many a woman. On the other hand, I've heard stories of women so petrified of being shamefully sent home because their contractions weren't real, they ignore some really important signs and barely make it to the hospital in time. A few clues about Braxton-Hicks contractions: They don't have a consistent pattern. They vary in length and strength and don't occur with regularity. Real contractions get longer and stronger and happen more frequently and at shorter intervals. The Braxton-Hicks also tend to occur mostly in one area, like the top of your uterus or the lower abdomen, whereas real contractions tend to radiate through your abdomen and lower back. And please don't let anyone tell you they don't hurt. They can absolutely hurt—I speak from experience. What people mean to say is that they don't hurt as much as the real thing. If you're concerned, don't be shy about calling your doctor.

Belly Button: In the strange but true department, your belly button may become particularly sensitive to the touch late in the third trimester. Your "inny" may now be an "outie." If you're already cursed with a severe outie like mine, pregnancy just makes it worse. My belly button, now well beyond button size, so more like a game show buzzer, was so huge my husband and I jokingly called it my third breast. It poked out through my clothes with reckless abandon and could have easily caused a puncture wound if anyone dared get close enough. If your navel is sensitive, protect it or press it down with a Band-Aid. My buzzer needed two large ones with an industrial strength adhesive—those cheaper brands just couldn't do the job.

Itchy Skin: Not only is your belly expanding beyond belief; it also itches like crazy. Some women find that something as simple as baby oil can help relieve the itchiness, while others need a concoction the thickness of the lard your grandmamma used to fry up her catfish. Leeza, from Dayton, Ohio, would get a big tub of real cocoa butter, add extravirgin olive oil, and with one of those paint mixing sticks, churn away. After whipping up a good batch, she says that stick came in handy to scratch places she could no longer reach.

If your itchiness turns into a rash that covers your tummy, butt, and thighs after the thirty-fifth week of pregnancy, you may be able to get some steroid creams that are safe to use and can take care of the problem; consult your doctor. Otherwise it will go away after you deliver.

Insomnia

Consider this bout of sleeplessness nature's way of preparing you for what lies ahead. With your big body and all the mental anxieties of soon-to-be mommyhood, it's no wonder you can't sleep. Not to mention that the activity in your stomach looks like you're the big tent of the UniverSoul Circus. As nature would have it, day-today activities like walking actually lull the baby to sleep, and when you're ready to sleep, she's now ready to get her party on! Unfortunately, it's not the last time you and your child's sleeping patterns will be at polar opposites. You may have heard advice to take a warm bath, drink a glass of warm milk, read a book, or meditate before going to bed. These are all great suggestions for you, but I've never heard anything on how to get that baby to stop doing the Humpty dance all night.

Swelling: Your growing baby makes it harder for blood to get to all the body parts that need it. That causes swelling in the legs, ankles, and feet. For some women the swelling is minor; for others ankles turn to cankles, shoes give way to flip-flops, and once-curvaceous legs become thick tree trunks. You should call your doctor if your entire body is swollen (poor dear!), if your legs are swollen at the beginning of the day, or if elevating your legs doesn't improve matters. Some other tips:

* Sleep on your left side at night. Experts say this position reduces the pressure on the veins that carry blood from the lower body back to the heart.
* Avoid tight socks, which can restrict your blood flow.
* Cut back your salt intake.
* Don't stand for long periods.
* Women who report no swelling of any sort were usually the ones who drank water as if they were dehydrated camels and took a brisk walk every day or so.

The Final Stretch

As a sister I must warn you that no matter how cute you've carried this pregnancy, and no matter how many people on the street tell you how good you look, there's a chance the time will arrive when it will be humanly impossible to be cute anymore. Try as you might, your feet and ankles will be too big, your face will be too distorted, your body will be too huge, your maternity clothes won't fit, or heaven help you, all of the above, to go anywhere or do anything. Even a statuesque beauty like Kimora Lee Simmons says there was a point when she stopped being seen in public (more from Kimora on page 237). Obviously, we all don't have the luxury to hibernate, but you're likely to want the most minimal amount of moving around and being seen by others. Your girlfriends may want a last night out. Not interested. Your husband may want a last quiet night of coziness. Get away from me; I will hurt you. And every mirror in your house will become a hated item.

Now, this is not true of all pregnant women. Sure, there are those who bounce through pregnancy, feeling happy and buoyant and comfortable all the way to the delivery room. Michelle Ebanks, group publisher of *Essence*, continued her weekly tennis matches with her husband all the way until one week before she delivered. "I never had that 'I can't take this anymore feeling,' " she says (hear more from Michelle on page 161. I say, more power to you! This is exactly the kind of woman we need commandeering the financial success of our most loved women's publication. But a good number of us will eventually get to the point when this pregnancy thing gets a bit tired and we're really ready for it all to be over—like right now, please. And that's okay. The way I see it, that's nature's way of getting you through delivery. Think about it; first, you dread delivery, and then pregnancy becomes so unbearable you actually wish for more hours of acute pain just to make the lingering discomfort go away. Do you see God's wisdom in all of this? And there, ladies, is your incentive to push.

In the meantime, try to stay relaxed. If you're comfortable, stay active. Do your best to look after yourself. I know you can't see your feet, but let somebody else massage them for you. Let your thoughts rest on your new baby—imagine his face, what your first words to him will be, whose features he'll have. You need the time to connect.

Nesting

Baby preparations including nursery and baby gear are probably also driving you mad. This is known as your nesting period—which sounds all warm and cozy, when what really happens is a lot more amped up and frenetic. In reality, think of it as your obsessive compulsive disorder nesting period, *OCDNP* for short. You *must* buy twelve more receiving blankets, now. You hate your sofa *now*. And every little photo frame provokes disgust. At some point, almost every partner will arrive home to find the furniture of some room completely rearranged, or find himself under hostile direct orders to move everything around quickly.

With my first child, I obsessed about everything in the nursery. I investigated every stroller, baby seat, bassinet, and high-chair combo known to man. And I bought every wipe, bottle, blanket, and food warmer on the market. If there was a breast warmer out there, I would have foolishly picked that up as well. Imagine a whole industry predicated on the concept that a baby should never feel anything cold, or even room temperature, for crying out loud. Ludicrous, to quote Mike. Meanwhile, on every madcap trip to Babies R Us, my mother would calmly tell me how I slept in a drawer for a few months, and that everything would be just fine without all the gadgetry. Of course, this only propelled my urge, as an overachieving black woman, to do so much better for my child. Besides, didn't they smoke and drink wine on the regular during pregnancy back then? I reminded my mom that she also didn't breast-feed me, and that that, along with the drawer thing, was surely grounds for a neonatal call to the Bureau of Child Welfare.

"I spent hours in the baby superstore, just meandering up and down the aisles collecting all the little doohickeys that I just *might* need down the road," remembers Roxanne, from Lithonia, Georgia. "My husband was no help. He's a gadget junkie anyway, so his usual electronic fixation was just transferred to baby stuff. I think he was worse than me," she says. As I did, Roxanne found those gadgets came in really handy—when other people had baby showers and we had several unopened packages to give away. Otherwise, they were pretty much completely useless. So, if you must nest, girls, nest responsibly. If you have the baby basics—blankets, diapers, undershirts, washcloths, bottles, and formula (if you're not breast-feeding), and a safe place for baby to sleep—you'll be fine.

Labor Plan

With all the focus on the pregnancy, it's a good time to think about and discuss with your doctor exactly how you want to get that baby out of your body, and to consider your preferences for pain relief and the possibility of a cesarean birth. Even if you're planning on not using any pain medication, you may want to know the choices just in case things become more difficult than you imagined. Sixty percent of the women I've met went into the hospital with one plan for their labor and delivery (candles, music, singing, no drugs) and went out with a completely different story (shouting, scream-ing, pooing on the table, getting an epidural). Says Denise, from Manassus, Virginia, "I was going to do the superwoman thing. 'I didn't need any drugs,' I said. After I got the epidural, I was like 'What was I thinking? This is great!' "

Your Baby

Around the seventh month your baby's lungs will produce a sub-stance that coats their lining. This helps your baby to use oxygen and helps the lungs stay open between breaths after birth. The baby's central nervous system is mature enough to sustain regular breathing outside the womb, and knowing that can be comforting to those concerned about preterm labor. A baby born after the twenty-seventh week has an 85 percent chance of survival, although there will likely be some problems.

By week twenty-six your baby is exploring his watery home and all the stuff in it, his eyebrows and eyelashes are well formed, and the footprints and fingerprints are also formed. Your baby may begin to recognize your voice, as well as your partner's, by week twenty-seven. It's hard for them to hear clearly since they still have a thick fatty protective coating covering their ears and all that amniotic fluid swishing around. By week twenty-eight, your baby's eyes, which have been sealed shut for the last few months to allow the retinas to develop, are beginning to open and close. Your baby will kick, no pun intended, into an accelerated growth spurt around the thirty-fifth week, gaining up to a half pound per week. And by the end of your ninth month, your baby weighs in at about six pounds or so and has likely already settled deeper into your pelvis in preparation for delivery (the baby can "drop" weeks before delivery or later, even the day labor begins).

By the start of your tenth month or week thirty-seven, your baby is considered full term. Even though he's got more growing to do, the rate of weight gain has slowed down a bit to about a half ounce a day. Even if his size isn't increasing dramatically, there are still staggering developments under way in the brain, nervous system, and other organs as their functions continue to improve. In the final three weeks, your baby's brain is tackling the complicated tasks of breathing, eating, digesting, and keeping the right heart rate. At forty weeks the average baby weighs about seven to eight pounds and is about eighteen to twenty and a half inches long. Babies of lesser or greater size can still be normal and healthy. And don't panic if your due date comes and goes without even a rumble from your little one. Only about 5 percent of women deliver on their due date. Stay positive and relaxed.

Your Job

Work life is likely becoming more and more difficult. The interrupted sleep, the commute, the difficulty concentrating and remembering things, the general discomfort and constant comments about your size and when you will deliver—it can be more than any procreating human can bear. As your maternity leave approaches, there may be added pressure from your boss, coworkers, or yourself to get matters organized, train other staff, update files, or take care of other things in preparation for your absence. You may also feel tempted to leave on a high note—close one last major deal, give one massive power presentation, snag one more new account, or create another office innovation—anything to leave one last impression of how valuable you are to the company. Sure, you can do these things, but don't think of them as job guarantees. And if it's stressing you out, you are doing harm to your pregnancy. At the end of the day, no matter what you do, you cannot control what happens in the office while you're gone. Your best defense is a good offense.

✳ Write a playbook. As early as possible put together a written job description, including a calendar with daily, weekly, and monthly duties. Include a step-by-step instruction guide, some helpful hints, along with client and contact information. Schedule a meeting with your boss to review all the preparations and plans for covering your duties. Offer work coverage solutions such as cross-training coworkers, junior employees, or colleagues in another department. Think outside the box when suggesting work coverage solutions—interns, temps, or recently retired employees who may still want to be active are all possibilities.

✳ If you're concerned that you will deliver early or be put on bed rest, write a condensed playbook focusing only on the most essential work that *must* be handled during your leave. Tell your boss how you'll get these top priorities covered and skip over the rest.

✳ The bigger and wobblier you get, the more your boss will be wondering whether you'll ever return to work. Use this time to reassure him constantly and emphasize the personal importance of your job. Speak positively of the future, and make references to things you are looking forward to (make them up if you have to!) when you return.

✳ Even if you've had a negative experience with your job and this pregnancy, try not to kick over a few wastepaper baskets on the way out. Leave on good terms. I know how some of us can be if someone crosses us—but don't sabotage the office; it can be self-defeating in the long run.

THE MOMENT OF TRUTH
Labor

Every mother has a labor story. And she has no problem telling you about it. You don't even have to ask. You don't even have to appear to be remotely interested. All she needs is a live body (comas apply) and she's off. You'll probably notice that a good majority of the ones that are always yapping about their labor experience have the most harrowing tale, complete with ear-cringing screaming, week-long labors, and seventy-two hours of straight pushing. Do not listen to these people. There are happy labor stories out there. Not happy in the hee, hee kind of way (there is a reason why they call it labor), but in the hee-hee-ho, hee-hee-ho, a few pushes and—is that it? kind of way. You can also listen to those who did have difficult birthing experiences but at least end their tale with a reminder of how amazing giving birth can be.

Still, as much as labor is the glue that binds all us mommies together, it is also a sticky issue. There's an unspoken rivalry between the women who delivered without pain medication and those who took a little nip from the epidural tap. The situation is about as bad as the supposed East Coast/West Coast rap thing.

Some women genuinely want the undiluted experience of childbirth. Others want just enough of the experience to guilt trip their husband and children for years to come, and then they want out. Those in the "no drugs" camp act as if someone stole the true meaning of giving birth by taking away the pain. Here's my rule: if a baby comes out of you, you're the real deal. For me, I'm not in labor for the pain. I'm a writer and it's all about the story. Once there's been enough of an experience for me to weave an engaging tale, I'm pretty much done.

Here's another thing I've noticed: we overachieving women have raised the bar on what "natural" childbirth is. Natural childbirth used to mean you delivered vaginally. Nowadays, it means you delivered vaginally *and* without any pain medication. Recently, a few moms were talking, and, of course, the labor stories started to roll. When one woman spoke of her "natural" birth and then mentioned an epidural, another woman butted in, "Well, that's not natural." Excuse me. Who changed the rules, and why wasn't I invited to the committee meeting? What's next—we'll have to break our own water, cut our own episiotomy, and deliver our own babies to make the "natural birth" cut? I don't think I like where this is headed. More importantly, women do not have to go into labor with something to prove. I think it's a really good idea to go to a childbirth class and learn about relaxation and breathing techniques, visualization and massage, among other strategies, but be open to other possibilities. Hard-and-fast rules don't always apply.

Whatever you do, make your own decisions. Keep in mind that it's hard to predict how *you* will actually feel in labor. Don't let anyone scare you into thinking you cannot do it without drugs. And don't let anyone make you feel any less than the phenomenal woman who you are because you took a hit in the back. Here, some of your sister friends who have been there, done that, share their labor stories, and their thoughts on the meds versus no meds flap:

One night I had contractions all night long, and then they stopped. I was frustrated and embarrassed. So the next night, when they started again, I was determined to ignore them until I was sure this was it. My husband and I were on the way to Copelands restaurant to get my favorite pasta dish—it has this cream sauce that I desperately craved. I was on a mission, but in pain. The contractions were coming faster and stronger. My husband says, "Do we need to turn around and go straight to the hospital?"

"NO!" I shouted.

But the contractions were getting worse. I agreed to get my pasta to go. I'm leaning against the bar, waiting for my food, and my husband, sensing that this was probably it, says to the bartender, "Let me get a beer and a shot." He continues, "I just need to take the edge off because I don't get an epidural." Meanwhile, the bartender is looking at both of us like we are crazy, as I'm bracing myself against the bar and my husband is throw-

ing back a shot. We made it to the hospital—my craving satisfied and my husband relaxed and our baby came that night. —Lorraine, Mableton, Georgia

Two weeks before my due date, we were told that the baby was very large. I was disappointed because we planned for a natural birth; we took the classes and everything. We were emotionally wrapped up in a natural birth. But when the doctor said there was a risk he could get stuck in the birth canal and they might have to pop his shoulder to get him out—I was like, okay, whatever is best for the baby. —Ivy, Saint Louis, Missouri

I got pregnancy-induced hypertension in my third trimester. It wasn't dangerous at first, but it had to be monitored. Two weeks before my due date I went to the doctor on my lunch break and my pressure was really high. My doctor said, "You have to stop working now. You're done. We're going to induce you tonight, before it affects the baby." I'll never forget it. It was a Friday. I couldn't believe this was happening. I kept thinking, this was supposed to happen naturally, I should go into labor. This is not how I envisioned giving birth.

I called my husband, went back to the office, and packed up a few things. My husband and I shifted into panic mode, but we were trying not to act it for fear of making the blood pressure worse. I didn't expect this sort of artificial, we're-going-to-have-to-induce, and your-baby's-birthday-is-tomorrow type of experience. Of all the physical things that I thought would happen, I never thought of this.

We went to the park and took pictures of me sitting, contemplating, and thinking. After our one hour of peace, quiet, and reflecting, we packed like crazy and went to the hospital.

I always hoped to have my baby naturally and without any pain medication. Maybe that was part of a fantasy that I would only feel slight discomfort. At the end I was realistic that I needed pain management. The epidural gave me the most peaceful rest. I actually slept for two hours; it was awesome. My baby girl came out with only fourteen minutes of pushing. There she was, five pounds, twelve ounces, and in great health. —Kuae, Montclair, New Jersey

I had my baby the way God intended, numb from the waist down. Those damn books make you think that if you just breathe, you'll be all right. Not for me. I had to put the book down and listen to my body. —Lisa, White Plains, New York

Mocha Mix: What the Sisters Say . . . About Your Mind, Body, Baby, and Job

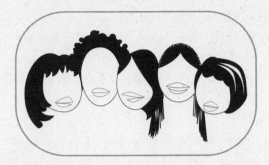

Your Mind

There's a lot to think about. How will I transition back to work? How do I sort out the financial issues, and the expense of child care? We don't live near our families, and looking into other options worries me. —Tanya, Ann Arbor, Michigan

The cycle of excitement and fear, of being amazed and humbled, of feeling great and feeling lousy—it's a ten month ride. —Tarsha, Detroit, Michigan

Your Body

I never knew pregnancy would take such a toll on my whole body. —Mya, Norfolk, Virginia

I had my first child at age twenty, and my second at age thirty-one and my body responded so drastically differently at thirty-one—it was unbelievable. —Janaris, Long Island, New York

Your Job

At work, it seemed there was little understanding that I was shepherding a life into the world. It was all about getting the maximum productivity out of you before you leave us high and dry. —Erica, Brooklyn, New York

I felt a lot of pressure at work. So much of my success or failure is hinged on the social aspects of the job, and I couldn't hang out in smoky bars and

restaurants with clients. I stopped flying for work in February and gave birth in March. When you're in a field with few women, you don't want to highlight that you are different. I was still fairly new to the job and needed to prove myself. You know, going to the bathroom constantly is not an option when you are tied to a trading screen. I tried to stay busy so I wouldn't feel the fatigue. I stood up while on the phone, because if I sat down it was over. In the end, I was limping to the finish line. —LISA, WHITE PLAINS, NEW YORK

You can't be clumsy when you're an accountant, and my mind was going. I had to triple check my work all the time. Also, my office is in the loft with a floor full of people below. Not only did I have the exhaustion of going up and down the stairs to get to the restroom, but everyone knew where I was going and how often. It was embarrassing. —DEBBIE, LOS ANGELES, CALIFORNIA

My workmates were very supportive. They brought in information they found on the Internet about what I should be doing and eating. Then they rigged something up underneath my desk so I could put my feet up. —SHERYL, STATEN ISLAND, NEW YORK

Your Baby
I remember sitting there crying about something or other, and then my baby kicked me for the first time. I stopped in the middle of my boo-hoo, and was like, was that my baby? Then I started crying tears of joy. After that, I never got tired of feeling him kick. —LAUREN, DALLAS, TEXAS

When you get down to the end, and you just don't think you can handle it much more. remember, the baby will come out. It has to. It is not a question. —LORRAINE, MABLETON, GEORGIA

The thought of body parts growing and forming inside of me was awesome. The fact that it was my job to provide the nutrients for these parts to grow properly was overwhelming. —JASMIN, PHOENIX, ARIZONA

Spotlight On . . .

Nicole Parker gave my mom and me one more thing to talk about. My mother loves the movie Remember the Titans. *So do I. But* Brown Sugar *was definitely a movie for my generation. And don't even think about calling my house on Wednesdays at 10:00 P.M. back when* Soul Food, *the series, was still on. The list of actresses that we both like is pretty short, but Nicole Parker is on both of them. And anyone who knows my mother can attest that this is no small feat. These days Nicole is going from the big screen to the big bump, and she landed a big hunk, Boris Kodjoe, as her partner in parenting baby Sophie Tei-Naaki Lee. Nicole is deeply rooted in holistic thinking and spiritual values—she did a body purification program, boosted Boris's sperm count, and closely investigated hypno-birthing.*

Boris and I wanted to have a family, but both had just come out of a relationship and we weren't rushing down the aisle. We tried for over a year to get pregnant and it didn't happen. When we were in Germany visiting Boris's family, he proposed, and then we went to Paris, and everything seemed so perfect, so right. On the way back, I was depressed because the trip was so romantic it would have been perfect if I was pregnant. I cried and cried. I was upset with God. I didn't understand why we were unable to conceive. Boris grabbed me and said, "This is our destiny to be parents. You can't stress yourself out, because it's going to be okay." So I called the doctor and I said, you know, I'm going to come in and investigate fertility options, and all of that stuff.

That next day, I went to the drugstore because my period was only spotting and I wanted to check. The test said I was pregnant, and I was so happy. I told Boris; he came home right away. He started shaking and he was sweating. Then he gave me the speech about I told you so, I told you so. When we went to the doctor, she said this baby was eleven days old. And when we counted back, we saw we'd conceived on the day he proposed. And that was June 20th, Father's Day.

I realize that it wasn't until God saw that we were ready to make this commitment that we were able to conceive. It's as if he was waiting for us to say, yes, you are my life partner. Ever since then, it has been a really magical time. Things that used to worry me don't matter anymore. I've released a lot of negativity and worries. I am making a baby and I just feel so blessed and special.

A few months prior to getting pregnant I did Queen Afua's cleansing and purification program. Her latest book, *Sacred Women*, is about getting your womb healed and your body together. I drank a lot of juices, and you really do feel like a new woman when you are done! After the cleansing, it's like every blessing came pouring down. I booked a film, Boris proposed, we found out I was going to have a baby, and then our new TV show got picked up. It was like, things were going really well. I was riding high spiritually, mentally, and physically.

My body was a clean slate for the baby to come in, and I'm sure that's why I didn't have one day of nausea. I did get severe fatigue and painful leg cramps in the middle of the night, from the instep of my foot all the way up to my hip. My doctor told me to increase my calcium.

The hair growth on my body, upper lip, and chin was out of control. I try to tweeze when I can, and the makeup lady on the show does a lot of it. Now that the show is on a break, I've got to figure out how to keep all of this together on my own. Boris doesn't let on that I'm a big hairy mess. He says that I'm beautiful, and that I'm glowing.

During my pregnancy I had a few emotional meltdowns over the smallest things. For example, one time I punched an address into the navigation system. Boris shut the car off. He knows it takes me a long time to punch in an address, letter by letter, and he turned the car off anyway and I had a meltdown. I was like, "You don't listen. I don't know if I can put my life in your hands." On top of that, he finished my water. So I said, "I'm carrying our baby and the baby needs water. You don't care. How could you drink it all?" I was tripping.

My plan going into labor is to be positive. Everybody has told me about the fat, tired, sick, evil, and the pain. I want to choose the positive. Instead of calling it labor, I call it birth. Even just changing the language can be calming. You can't have ten months of fear. I investigated hypno-birthing, which focuses on deep relaxation and trusting that your body has everything it needs to give birth. They claim you can get into a state of calm where you release your own sedative, your own pain medicine, and have a pain-free birth. On the tapes, you see women breathing deeply and the baby just slides out. I went to see it for myself. I was all up in a bunch of ladies' business. It was no joke. That's what I'm working on.

A lot of black women don't understand that certain foods and products have a different reaction in our body. We shouldn't be drinking coffee or Coke or even chewing gum. It all has stuff that affects our ovaries. So many black women are trying to get pregnant and they don't even consider the diet. You don't think it affects your colon, womb, uterus, or ovaries. But that stuff will eat you up inside.

An herbalist named Djehuty Maat'ra educated me about black women and their womb and taught Boris about his sperm count. A lot of black men are athletes and don't realize that spending too much time in basketball shorts or in the hot tub can kill your sperm count. These are things that men shouldn't do. He tripled Boris's sperm count. Not to mention his sex drive. I told him, "I'm going to have to get you a girlfriend. There is only so much one person can do."

The best advice is that you can choose your own kind of pregnancy. You can choose peace. You can choose relaxation. You can choose it to be pain free. And when you engage your mind in that direction, it is the most wonderful experience. Of course, I am not going to suffer. But I'm going to go into it fully confident, at peace and without fear, yet open to improvise if I need to.

ReTell Therapy

THE QUEEN OF THE C

by Katrina Ruiz

I am the C-section queen. My reign began with my first pregnancy, when after countless hours of being in labor my obstetrician simply said, "You're just not a big girl on the inside." With that said, he then put me under anesthesia and when I woke up, I had a beautiful girl named Autumn. The joy from my new baby was totally eclipsed by my recovery. As soon as the anesthesia wore off, there were nurses all around me ordering me to get out of the bed and walk around. Didn't they know that I just had my abdomen cut open, sewn back together, and then stapled! This was all a bit overwhelming. I couldn't laugh without fear that I would bust a stitch. Picking up and holding my baby were also difficult. I soon learned that the key to recovery from a cesarean section is optimal pain management, i.e., drugs.

During my stay in the hospital, it was easy to figure out which mothers had vaginal births and which ones had cesarean births. The C-section moms moved in slow motion, holding their midparts, while the vaginal birth moms sprinted down the hallway. When I left the hospital I was ordered not to take baths, drive, or go up and down the stairs for several weeks. I later learned that the medical term for my narrow insides is *cephalopelvic disproportion*. I was determined to relinquish my crown for my subsequent pregnancies.

Five years later, I became pregnant with my second child. My doctor, husband, and I were optimistic that I could successfully have a VBAC [vaginal birth after cesarean] delivery. We even took the classes. The baby, however, had another plan. After several hours, the same doctor who delivered my first baby crushed my VBAC dreams and cut me open. This time I had an epidural instead of being gassed. I was awake, with my husband by my side, for the whole delivery. The recovery after my baby girl was much better.

Five years passed and I became pregnant again. A sonogram confirmed that this baby was a big boy. My obstetrician figured that—based on my history—it was highly unlikely, if not impossible, for me to deliver this baby vaginally. She then presented me with the new millennium option—a scheduled C-section. Typically, they wait until you are close to your due date and then you pick a day to come in and have your baby. How convenient! No long hours in labor, no exceeding the speeding limit trying to get to the hospital, no pesky fluid sacs breaking at the wrong time. What a great idea! But having a spinal block really concerned me. After doing some research I decided to go with it. The doctor and I coordinated our schedules—we were both free on December 12. My husband and I arrived at the hospital stress-free. I actually walked into the delivery room. About thirty minutes later, my beautiful eight-pound son named Jonathan was born.

A scheduled C-section is convenient and virtually painless, but not body-friendly. Going into labor tells your body to get ready for a series of events, but my body got no such messages. My breast milk took a long time to come in and my hormones were off for months. In retrospect, I would have definitely preferred to go into labor and then have the surgery.

No matter how my children got here, I am so glad they are here. My recoveries from the C-sections were challenging but only temporary. Being with my children and watching them grow make it all worthwhile.

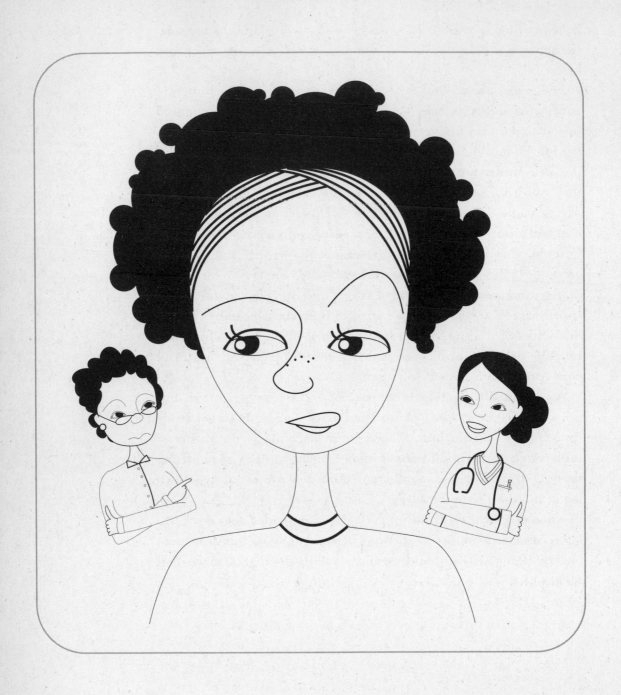

3

Truth Versus Lies

The Real Deal on
Ten Common Pregnancy Myths

Before these nine months are over, a number of women, most likely your mama, your grandmother, or their friends, will tell you a number of things about what you should or should not do during pregnancy. They will also tell you how they are categorically sure of the sex of your baby. Throughout both of my pregnancies my mother kept telling me not to raise my hands up over my head because it would get the umbilical cord stuck around the baby's neck. She was so adamant about it, she made me paranoid. I made my husband empty all the kitchen cabinets and put everything on the counter, just in case I needed something and nobody was around to reach it for me. Everyone who came by thought we just had an exterminator come in. And what about raising just one hand? Was that dangerous? By the time I got into my third trimester I wouldn't reach up, down, or to the side, for anything. My husband got so tired of my asking him to pass me stuff at the dinner table, he would routinely place salt, pepper, beverages, salad dressing, hot sauce, or all other necessary (and unnecessary) condiments in a neat circle directly around the rim of my plate.

The point is, all of this drama was caused by my mother—more specifically, her insistence on this don't-raise-your-hands-over-your-head law. It was not until doing the research for this book that I realized that that is an old wives' tale. When I confronted my mom about this, she shrugged and said, "Old wives' tale? Maybe. But better safe than sorry." Was that the best she could do? She has no idea of what I subjected myself to, believing that she spoke from medical facts. And my poor husband, if he finds out, I'm dead.

I'm sure my mom is not the only person scaring the bejesus out of unsuspecting pregnant women with old wives' tales deftly disguised as medical truths, or giving women false hopes on the gender of their babies based on ancient rituals. These things have been a part of black folks' culture for a long time. Many of the old wives' tales date back to slavery, when we didn't have access to proper medical attention and simply relied on other women to get us through pregnancy and childbirth. This word-of-mouth advice from old wives' tales to cure-all remedies was passed on from generation to generation; some of these beliefs even originated in the traditions of certain African tribes. The good news is that this oral history has been preserved to this day with many of these age-old beliefs still lingering among modern day folks. But it's hard to figure out what's true or false when your mother, grandmothers, and aunties plead such a convincing case. To help get a handle on these tales I've compiled a list of ten common pregnancy myths, and then I let the sisters and the medical lot weigh in.

Myth 1: You'll strangle the baby with its umbilical cord if you reach up over your head.

What I Say: Now that I know that it's just a wives' tale, I can knock down a few notches of neuroticism, but I can't say I would completely ignore this one. For me, it falls into that stretch mark kind of category. Sure, they say you can't prevent them and it's all about genetics, but why risk it, especially if you're in a high-risk pregnancy. Besides, do you know what happened the last time I tried to prove my mama wrong?

What the Mocha Mix Says: My unofficial survey agrees: it is probably an old wives' tale, but few were willing to risk it. Besides, how can you argue against getting people to do more things for you while you're pregnant? Bottom line: reach only when no one else can do it or it's absolutely necessary—like the time when some cruel person put the chocolate syrup on the top shelf.

What the Experts Say: Doctors say this absolutely is an old wives' tale. Movements of your extremities have nothing to do with the baby's umbilical cord, they say. In fact, according to one study involving one thousand consecutive deliveries, more than 20 percent had a cord around the neck and there were no deaths. This is apparently pretty common. And it is an absolute rarity to have a cord become so tight that it stops blood flow and causes death. In cases when this does happen, doctors say that such "cord accidents" are impossible to prevent.

Myth 2: Don't chemically relax or color your hair when pregnant.

What I Say: I tried to hold off as long as possible, avoiding a relaxer just in case it wasn't safe in the first trimester. One day I woke up and my hair looked like I had just been rolling down the river with Ike, and I could wait no more. As far as I am concerned, it's a lot healthier for me to look good and, ergo, feel good about myself than it is for me to look like a black Chia Pet and be depressed. And what's good for me has to be good for baby, right?

Also, the chemicals of a relaxer don't worry me as much as all the smells of the hairdresser—burning hair, sheens and sprays, and the haze of blow drying. Have you ever been in the salon and you can barely see the front door because of all the smoke coming off the blow dryers? I couldn't bear the thought of being confined someplace with no fresh air. So, if I had to wait in between a conditioning treatment, or a blow, I would wait outside. I would also try to go to the salon early in the morning, when there were fewer people and fewer fumes.

By the time my second pregnancy came around, I got highlights in my second trimester and didn't even think twice. But I always hit the salon early in the day before the crowd and the smells picked up.

What the Mocha Mix Says: Some women tried to get a relaxer less frequently during their pregnancy, trying to stretch it out eight or nine weeks, for example, instead of their customary four- to six-week visit. For Stephanie from Washington, D.C., not getting a relaxer was not even an option. "Oh, hell no! I'd just have to pop an extra prenatal vitamin, drink an extra glass of milk, or something else to toughen up my baby, but I was most definitely keeping the do intact," she says.

What the Experts Say: Various studies on humans and animals show that only a very small amount of anything applied to your scalp is actually absorbed into your system, and therefore little is able to reach your developing baby. Low levels of hair dye can be absorbed through the skin and excreted through the urine, but this minimal amount is not thought to be of harm to the baby, according to the findings. Basically the data haven't shown there to be any adverse effects on your pregnancy. Some doctors are still split on this issue. Talk to your doctor; she may likely just recommend waiting until you're in the second trimester, just to be safe.

A cautionary note to our sister stylists: a landmark study of reproductive disorders among hairdressers, based on a sample from Baltimore, Maryland, showed a slightly increased risk of miscarriage among cosmetologists with specific work patterns. Those activities included a workweek of more than forty hours, standing for more than eight hours a day, higher numbers of bleaches and perms applied per week, and working in a salon where nails are also done. Later studies showed a slightly decreased risk, perhaps due to better working conditions and newer restrictions on some dye formulas, but both studies support the importance of proper working conditions for hair professionals. Working in a well-ventilated area, wearing protective gloves, taking frequent breaks, and avoiding eating and drinking in the workplace were listed as significant factors that can decrease risk.

Myth 3: Stuff chilled collard greens or cabbage leaves in your bra to soothe sore breasts.

What I Say: Now I hadn't even heard this one before embarking on the journey of this book, but apparently women swear by it. I found a lot of information that the cabbage actually works but there wasn't much info on the collard greens. I'm sure that's just black folks' improvising on a mainstream idea, and collards work just as well. Much of the research focused on using the cabbage for breast-feeding moms who are sore from engorged breasts, but a lot of women said it helped with the soreness of pregnancy boobs as well. My only question is, If these chilled leaves are such a magical cure-all for soreness, why can't we use them on our aching back, legs, shoulders, arms, pelvis?

What the Mocha Mix Says: Go ahead! Stuff your bra with cabbage or collards for some relief. What the heck, throw in a ham hock for flavor, too! "My mama told me that a long time ago," Audrey, from Columbia, South Carolina, says. "And I'm never pregnant or nursing without some cabbage in the fridge!"

What the Experts Say: It's true. There's apparently some chemical or combination of chemicals within the leaf that soothes the breast and inhibits engorgement. This leaf remedy is so well known (where have I been?) that a doctor even studied it. In 1993 some doctor took one hundred and twenty breast-feeding women seventy-two hours after delivery and put them into two groups. One group was treated with cabbage leaves and the other group received the routine care. The women with cabbage-stuffed bras breast-fed longer and had greater success. Another doctor studied the effect of a chilled leaf versus one that is room temperature. That test was inconclusive as both groups of women reported less pain after a two-hour period. So, either way it works. But it does seem like common sense that anything cold is more likely to help reduce pain and swelling. Now that you know it works, don't just go stuffing leafy veggies in your bra willy-nilly. There's apparently a science to this cabbage or collard thing. Here it is: cut out the thick stem and cover your breast with cold leaves, stem end down. Leave the nipple uncovered. Change the leaf when the leaf goes limp. Stop as soon as your breasts feel comfortable.

Myth 4: If you deny yourself a particular craving, your baby's birth-mark will have that shape.

What I Say: Sounds like a bunch of hooey to me. That is, until my son was born and I noticed that if you flip him upside down and tilt him at a thirty-two-degree angle, his birthmark looks just like a bottle of Hypnotiq—exactly what I really needed to get through that pregnancy. My daughter has a nearly perfect circle of a birth-mark, about the size of a quarter. Does this mean my craving for money during my pregnancy was denied? Could be.

What the Mocha Mix Says: For every woman who tossed this one off as nonsense, there was someone who heard a story or personally experienced something that made it true. Mischelle, from Jackson-ville, Florida, said she craved red pasta sauce and strawberries all the time but tried not to indulge as often as she really wanted to. Her daughter was born with a red blotch on her back.

What the Experts Say: Hooey.

Myth 5: A little swig of castor oil can help bring on labor.

What I Say: I am not a fan of anything that makes me lose control of my bodily functions. My problem with this one is that, while castor oil may bring on the labor, it can also bring on a bad case of the runs. Apparently castor oil—interestingly, it's oil from the seed of a large African plant—is powerful stuff. My grandmother says the key is to have just the right amount to help your contractions but not unleash the gates of your bowels. However, if I'm miserable and overdue, I don't think it's the best time to start playing mad scientist. Besides, something that opens the floodgates of your bowels doesn't necessarily do the same for your uterus—it's a completely different body system, people! When you weigh the risk of possibly releasing your bowels all over the delivery table versus sticking it out one more day, I'll go for another marathon walk in the mall, thankyouverymuch.

What the Mocha Mix Says: Some women still say this worked for them. Of course, there's always the element of coincidence. Leila, from Trenton, New Jersey, said she was absolutely miserable and "ready to reach in and yank the baby out myself." She tried a tablespoon of castor oil and went into labor three hours later. Audrey, from Illinois, reports the same. She was four days overdue and took a tablespoon of castor oil before she went to bed. She was awakened by labor pains six hours later (forget the castor oil, how did she sleep for six hours straight at that stage?). Bottom line: you can try it if you like, but be prepared to deal with its other effects.

What the Experts Say: Completely false. One doctor pointed me to a study from the *South African Medical Journal* back in 1987. Not only did the women in this group have ridiculous diarrhea but apparently so did the babies. They found that babies born to women who took a hit of castor oil before labor had a greater incidence of meconium-stained amniotic fluid. Meconium is the greenish fluid that is produced when the baby has a bowel movement in its amniotic sac. Fetal respiratory problems can result if the baby inhales this fluid at delivery.

Myth 6: I know it's a boy because . . . I know it's a girl because . . .

What I Say: I will bet a lot of money that before your pregnancy is over, a gazillion people, most of whom are complete strangers, will go up to you—size up the shape of your belly, your physical appearance, or the way you walk—and tell you whether you're carrying a boy or a girl. When you're pregnant, everyone has a gender guess. Some people say carrying low is a boy and carrying high is a girl. Others call it vice versa. It's fun to play along, but after a while, it can get a bit annoying when all you want to do is grab your pint of vanilla Swiss almond Häagen-Dazs and get back to your comfy sofa instead of being bombarded by a hundred old ladies on the way out of the store.

What the Mocha Mix Says: Here are a few of the favorites from women across the country:

* If it's a boy, you carry high and round. If it's a girl, you carry low (or vice versa, depending on the person you ask).
* If you're still looking good, it's a boy. Boys preserve your looks. Girls steal your beauty.
* To find out what you're having, thread a needle and hold it over a pregnant woman's stomach. If the needle moves from side to side, it's a boy. If it moves up and down, it's a girl. I've also heard a variation on this: you put the woman's wedding ring on a string and do the same thing.
* Eat a clove of garlic. If the smell seeps out of your pores, it's a boy. If the smell isn't detected at all, it's a girl.
* If you have a lot of acne, it's a girl. And brewing all those extra hormones for a female is what is affecting your skin.
* If you trip or fall over your own feet during pregnancy, it's a boy. If you're graceful, it's a girl.

✳ There's the old Draino test. This one is not from African Americans per se, but it's strange enough to mention. Here's how it works: pee in a glass jar with some Drano in it. If the mixture is green, it's a girl. If it's blue, it's a boy.

✳ This one isn't African American either, but it is native American—close enough. As my girl Joyce says, "If you brown, you down." The Mayans determined the sex of the baby by taking the mother's age at conception and the actual calendar year of conception. If both are even or odd, it's a girl. If one is even and one odd, it's a boy.

What the Experts Say: I couldn't find one to comment on these wives' tales. It's all hooey to them.

Myth 7: Don't go to a funeral or look at a dead person, or your baby will have some feature of that person.

What I Say: I don't know about picking up a dead person's nose or chin, but admittedly, going to funerals freaks me out when pregnant. I know this for sure because I went to a funeral when I was about eight months pregnant. I was just trying to be supportive of my auntie, who had lost someone close to her. My mother and father told me not to go. But I'm stubborn, even when gestating. So I went. And there was something about all the flowers, the crying, the slow grind of the organ music, and the singing that totally freaked me out. I didn't want my baby to hear any songs of sorrow. I didn't want my baby to hear any outbursts of grief. As any mother does, you want your baby to be surrounded by tranquillity and happiness—there'll be enough drama in the real world when he gets out. I couldn't bear it for very long. So I blamed it on the uncomfortable pews and waited outside. Afterward I had terrible dreams about death for about a week. All in all, it was a bad experience. I really wished I had listened to my mother (she's going to enjoy reading that line!).

What the Mocha Mix Says: Most women said the dearly deceased had to be high up on the family food chain to get them into a funeral. Considering how emotional most black folks' funerals can get, most women said it was a bit more than they could handle. I didn't find anyone who said she saw a dead person and her baby showed up sporting his or her dimples. Bottom line: hooey but perhaps not worth the emotional stress.

What the Experts Say: Double hooey.

Myth 8: If you have a small shoe size, you will have a C-section.

What I Say: Off the bat, this one could apply to me. Before my children made my feet grow like the Jolly Green Giant, I had been a size six or six and a half for years. And I've had two C-sections. I'm up to a seven and a half now. But my sister has always had ample feet, she's a size nine, and she's had three C-sections.

What the Mocha Mix Says: This one was mixed fifty-fifty. Of the women that I spoke to who had C-sections, almost half of them wore a shoe size of seven and a half or less. So there may be something to this one. There was also a size eleven woman in Michigan (she begged for me not to reveal her name) who's had two C-sections, so go figure.

What the Experts Say: After speaking to a few doctors, I think this one may have some roots in medical science. The idea is that those smaller feet are usually attached to smaller women, and petite women do have a higher cesarean rate. That's because these women tend to have smaller pelvic bones, and since they don't necessarily have smaller babies, their kids get stuck more often. One study in Britain sampled three hundred fifty-one women. Fifty-seven of these women had a shoe size of less than four and a half (U.S. size six and a half) and an overall cesarean rate of 21 percent. A second group with a shoe size between four and a half and six (U.S. six and a half to eight) had a 10 percent cesarean rate, and a third group with sizes greater than six (U.S. size eight) had a 1 percent rate. So this study did find a correlation between small shoe size and increased C-section rate. Another study found no connection between shoe size and section rate but found a significantly higher rate in women less than five feet two inches in height.

Back in the States, a few doctors said these British studies made interesting reading but no clinical difference. In fact, there are plenty of us shorties out there delivering vaginally and plenty of Big Foots getting the horizontal cut.

Myth 9: Don't lie flat or sleep on your back.

What I Say: As you know or will soon find out, pregnancy limits your sleeping position options. Sleeping on your stomach after about two and half months is out. And now they want to take away sleeping on my back. That means an easy six months of lying on your side only, which to me is tantamount to cruel and unusual punishment. If I woke up and had inadvertently rolled over on my back, I'd worry that I might have done some serious damage. Here's the medical rationale for the no sleeping on the back rule: you probably know by now, your uterus sits in the center of the pelvis. As it gets larger during your pregnancy it eventually takes up the entire lower abdomen. When this happens, the uterus is lying directly over a large vein called the *vena cava,* a very important vein, which carries all the oxygen-poor blood from the lower half of the body back to the heart and lungs to be reoxygenated and pumped out again to the rest of the body. As the uterus gets bigger, it puts pressure on the vena cava, which can limit blood flow back to the heart. So, if a pregnant woman lies directly on her back, the uterus squashes the vena cava against the backbone and there is less blood available to be pumped out to the placenta, and that can basically frustrate a growing baby. But before you panic, check out what the doctors have to say.

What the Mocha Mix Says: "This one really freaked me out," says Tonya, of Raleigh-Durham, North Carolina. "I kept wondering if there was a time expiration on that. I mean, can I take a power nap on my back or was it full-fledged sleeping that will do you in?" And if sleeping on your back is a no-no, what about other things you do on your back? "Every now and then my husband would, you know, take a trip down South, as they say, to make a sister feel good. But I really couldn't enjoy it because I kept worrying that I was going to hurt the poor baby. Then I was trying to rush him and you can't rush that, and we tried a chair or the edge of the bed, but nothing really worked out. Come to think of it, I really gave up a lot for that baby!" recalls Sheena, from Memphis, Tennessee.

What the Experts Say: As doctors explained it to me, the body has its own ways of protecting itself. For example, you can try to hold your breath forever, but basically you'll pass out, your body will automatically take over, and you'll regain normal breathing patterns. Such is also the case with a woman who is preggers. If she does squash the vena cava significantly enough to decrease blood flow to the baby, then other things like your brain won't be getting enough blood either. At this point, as one doctor put it, "Your brain sends you a complex signal, like, 'Roll over, stupid; this doesn't feel too good,' and sure enough you wake up and roll over onto your side." My doctor said not to panic if you wake up and find yourself on your back. You have not cut off junior's blood supply. Just roll over to your side and go back to sleep.

Myth 10: Pregnant women crave dirt and clay.

What I Say: I think you have to be from the deep, deep Deep South to know about this one, but apparently there are women who crave dirt and/or red clay while pregnant. This practice of clay eating (technically called *geophagy* or *pica*) originated in some West African tribes (the people who became most of the North American slaves) and is said to be a response to a physiological need for calcium and minerals, particularly of pregnant or lactating women. Others say it was just a common craving among black women. At one point, historians say, plantation owners devised mouth locks to prevent slaves from eating dirt. It's not just an African thing either. Plato wrote about Greek women who ate soil, and the Swedes used to add clay to their flour when making bread, according to one professor. Here's the yummy part—some of these dirts are "mined" from termite mounds or other nutrient-rich areas and sold at the local gas station or general store. Women bake it in the oven for a few hours and then season it with vinegar and salt or fry it up with a little grease. This practice persists in the rural South, especially in parts of eastern Alabama.

What the Mocha Mix Says: The responses ranged from a freaked-out "What type of foolishness is that?" to a very calm "Oh yeah, I heard about that from my grandmother."

What the Experts Say: It's a shame, but these days not even dirt is what it used to be. Poisons from manufacturing plants, and contaminants such as pesticides, seep into the soil, leaving a high potential of contamination for today's dirt eaters. Even Alabama's state toxicologist has warned against dirt eating because of the contaminants and for other reasons. In general, eating dirt or starch is a no-no—doctor's orders.

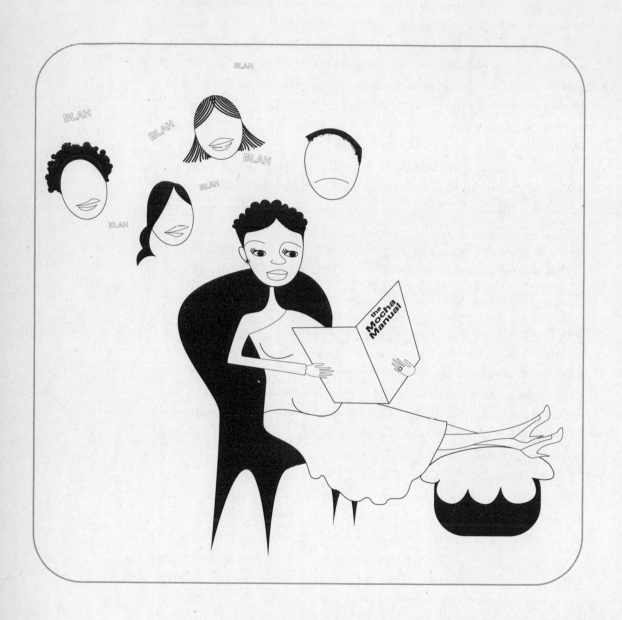

4

Pregnancy and Your Peeps

FROM YOUR GIRLFRIENDS TO YOUR PARTNER—YOUR RELATIONSHIPS ARE ABOUT TO CHANGE

GIRLFRIENDS

Every girl needs her sister fix. Whether they are from your old neighborhood, sorority, church, college, or work, we all have a sister circle. From the man troubles, money troubles, family troubles, office politics, health issues, weddings, funerals, interventions, to that three-month funk you were in—your girlfriends have been there through it all. So you may have just envisioned your pregnancy as simply another thing for you and your girls to share. That sounds lovely, but don't be surprised if it doesn't work out that way. Chances are, pregnancy will change the nature of your relationship with your girlfriends, especially if you're one of the first in your circle to become pregnant. You see, pregnancy is a strange situation.

First of all, you're probably starting to separate emotionally from your previous carefree childless life, and your girlfriends are a big part of that life. Second, yes, your girls love you, but not even your closest girlfriend wants to hear the latest update on your bout with projectile vomiting, and even your dearest friend might be ready to kick you to the curb when those pregnancy hormones make you an emotional train wreck. If there ever was a test of a friendship, it wasn't that obnoxious guy with the annoying snorting laugh you dated in college, even though your girls hated him: it is pregnancy.

Remember: pregnancy is a ten-month diversion from your usual self. And just because your girls can't get enough of you with an empty uterus, that doesn't mean they'll be head over heels for you with surging hormones and swollen limbs. So don't be surprised if there's a little less love going on. You may even feel that you guys have less and less in common these days, particularly when they want a girls' night out and you want to relax at home with a stack of parenting books. And besides, why would anyone want you around? You're hormonal. You can't drink. You shouldn't hang out in smoky clubs and bars, the slightest smells spark dizzy spells, and however exciting it may sound to you, nobody wants to meet you at the gym for prenatal aerobics. And they don't want to hear your endless supply of fascinating fetal development facts—"Guess what, my baby got a pancreas six hours ago, and in seventy-two hours he will blink for the first time." Face it; you are not the girlfriend you used to be.

Given these changed circumstances, it's no wonder the world of expecting women is littered with stories of girlfriends who stopped calling because they knew you would turn down another invite because of exhaustion. For some, it's a slow drift—the calls slowly decrease from every day to once a week, to once a month, to see-ya-when-I-see-ya. "I can't remember the point when the calls actually ended. But my friends just eventually stopped inviting me out," says Phyllis from Chicago. Other women say the cut was swift. But being an extremist, and a perfectionist laced with a fear of failing at anything in my life, I went overboard in the opposite direction. I was determined not to let pregnancy ruin my friendships, to have some fragment of a social life, and to try to go on kicking it with my girls', big belly and all. So, off we went one night to a private party. It was a nonsmoking venue, so I felt safe. And I was looking cute—rockin' some knee-high black boots with a three-inch heel, sippin on my ginger ale with extra cherries. I was sitting around gloating like, yeah, this is how you do pregnancy. But as the night wore on, I remembered that my pregnancy tolerance for high heel shoes is roughly about 17.4 minutes, and I was secretly craving my ugly comfortable shoes with the fleece lining. Then I became acutely aware of the music, which seemed to have become really loud all of a sudden, and I began to feel guilty. It didn't stop there. Superparanoia set in and I feared my baby was going to be deaf from all of this loud thumping, and in my panic I saw vivid images of the vibrations of sound rising through the floor somehow, sending me into premature labor. To make matters worse, if I showed up at the hospital in these boots, I would certainly be stereotypically mistaken for a hoochie with no health insurance and I would be left on a gurney in the hallway to die, or worse, deliver my baby myself. Or so I thought. I was a nervous wreck. On the other side, I didn't want to be the pregnant party pooper. My friends seemed so happy that we were all out, I didn't want to tell them I was having a psycho pregnant woman moment complete with chronic foot pain and delusions. Besides, when you're pregnant you are automatically the designated driver. So I took a time out in the bathroom. I sat on a toilet seat in hysteria for about an hour, trying my best to chill out. That night was my last night out with the girls.

You're a different person now, and your friends who've never been pregnant may not understand this new you. And no matter how much you try to explain what it feels like to be pregnant, your childless girlfriends will never really understand. Call it the mommy divide. It's bigger than the digital divide, wage gap, male/female communication gap, and Grand Canyon put together, and it unites women who are pregnant or have children and divides them from women who don't. But don't fret. In his supreme wisdom, the giver of life creates a new place for you to share, expound on, and be comforted by. You are a rightful member of a fresh, new, therapeutic forum that has now opened up to you and will be all that your girlfriends cannot be. That forum is made up of complete and total strangers who are also pregnant. For some unknown reason, yet to be determined by medical science, pregnancy brings about a strong urge to talk to other pregnant women. And even if you're an angry black woman on the edge, you'll find yourself smiling at or talking to total strangers in the frozen food aisle of the grocery store just because they're pregnant, too. You'll ask these strangers personal and intimate questions; you'll compare belly sizes, compare swollen limbs, and talk about food cravings in a way that borders on eroticism. These are the things your girl-friends just won't understand. It's strange, but now you are part of the unspoken sisterhood of procreators, and your old girlfriends with their yet unstretched uteruses, and their jeans that still fit, just won't do it for you at times.

The best advice is to let it happen. You're just going to end up hating them or playa hatin' them anyway, with their designer out-fits and showing off their tone bodies while they sip on colorful cocktails—while your butt is spreading like jam and you're about ready to give your right arm for a highly caffeinated cup of coffee.

Most of us are blessed with a few friends who will stick it out with us. And remember they are adjusting to a new situation, too. I had a girlfriend who would begin every conversation with a drawn out "Hoooow—are—you—feeling?" It was very slow and enunciated as if pregnancy wipes away English as your first language or turns you into a retard. Boy, was that annoying. But I knew she was just try-ing her best. Also, don't always take that "How are you?" question so literally. You're thinking, oh, that's my girl right there asking about my well-being. The honest truth is they don't really care. They are just checking in to make sure you haven't stopped breath-ing, tripped, killed your husband, or blown up your workplace—all of which are very real possibilities for a pregnant black woman. Do not take this opportunity to tell them how many times you peed today or how you ate two chili cheese hot dogs with hot sauce and salsa for lunch. "My friends later told me that I drove them crazy with all the pregnancy information," says Deidre, from Jonesboro, Arkansas.

Divulging too many details is potentially defeatist to you. Let me explain. All circles of girlfriends have the same next-generation fantasy: You know, the one when we all meet the man of our dreams around the same time, then we all have fabulous to-die-for weddings in succession, then we all get pregnant together and our children grow up together. Our children become best friends or marry each other and, of course, as our offspring spend countless hours talking about what cool parents we are. We, in turn, will share almost all of our embarrassing moments and drama escapades with them while sitting around sipping hot cocoa in front of the fireplace. It's like a Kodak moment, Disneyworld commercial, and *Soul Food* (the TV series) all rolled up into one.

But sometimes too much information can send your friends running in the opposite direction. I made the mistake of sharing too many gory details of pregnancy with a close friend, a friend I was heavily recruiting to join the mommy hood. Instead, I traumatized the poor woman and sent her running scared from even the mere thought of pregnancy. Too much sharing with childless friends that you want to have children in the future may be counterproductive. Share in good measure, but don't shoot yourself in the foot.

And don't throw your single or childless friends away. They have a very important role to play. Likely, they will be the ones to plan your baby shower. This is a crucial job. You know your other friends with kids don't have time to plan a meal, let alone a baby shower fabulous enough for your firstborn. So be kind to them. There's also a better chance they will help you out when you're on the mend and have a new baby.

In the meantime be prepared for girlfriends to turn into all sorts of different personalities. They tend to fall into certain categories, with each taking on a distinct positive or negative role in your pregnancy production. After speaking to many of your sister friends, here's a sampling of what you can expect from your girlfriends when you're expecting.

Girlfriend Type One

Almost every woman has a girlfriend she will describe as the one she "couldn't have made it through without." These are treasured friends, and they may not be the same person all the time, or one person, for that matter. I couldn't have survived at work without Cora. My girlfriend Sherese was my endless listening ear and spiritual adviser. Keiva lives closest, so she would do the physical check-ins, grocery pickups, and other errands for me. And Schalawn, my partner in high-end indulgences and the undisputed Los Angeles queen of exfoliating and moisturizing, would send me care packages with lots of bath salts and body oils. I gotta admit, it was the best. But what really made my girls so indispensable is that they always told me how good I looked. Basically, they were good liars. When I cried about how fat I was, they would all vehemently deny it and tell me I didn't even look pregnant from the back: lie. When I whined about my puffy face with matching nose, they insisted it wasn't that bad at all: another lie. But this is why you have friends, to tell you the lies that help you get through and to tell you the truth only when you're about to embarrass yourself. These are the blessings of girlfriends. Pray you will have one of these.

Girlfriend Type Two

This type always want to treat you to lunch, treat you to pizza, or treat you to a pedicure. Basically, they have so little understanding of what you're going through or they feel so bad for you that they resort to throwing money at you. It's pity money, but do take it anyway. After all, you've got to save all your extra pennies for junior's baby gear and college fund. Treaters don't usually expect anything in return, and this is how they try to be supportive.

Girlfriend Type Three

These friends are so ridiculously clueless about anything related to pregnancy that they keep inviting you to the club, wine tasting parties, skiing—all the things you can't do, as if you're just growing a watermelon under your shirt. Naomi, from Augusta, Georgia, says her friends were "buggin' out" because she stopped going to their weekly Happy Hour ritual. "They couldn't understand that I just wasn't into that scene anymore," she says. "I just had no interest." These friends are also the type who call and interrupt your sleep, and instead of recognizing how precious sleep is to a pregnant woman and calling back later, they drone on as if they never heard you say you were sleeping. They mean no malice. Calmly explain to them all the things you won't be doing for at least the next few months, and tell them of your new bedtime. If that doesn't work, just wait until your third trimester. You'll likely be up in the middle of the night anyway because you're too uncomfortable to sleep; then call them at 3:00 A.M. and act equally oblivious to the fact that they were probably enjoying some serious z's.

Girlfriend Type Four

Any psychologist will tell you that it's very common for women actually to be jealous of their childbearing friends—particularly if you're the first in the crew to conceive or your friends have not married yet. Sometimes these friends engage in rude and insensitive comments such as, "Look how fat you are!" or "Are you supposed to be that big?" or, my personal favorite, "Are you going to eat another one of those?"—the answers to the latter two being yes and yes. Or they may be judgmental about your pregnancy choices or keep talking about how painful childbirth will be. Just ignore these people.

In any situation, if you find that one of your girls is intentionally or unintentionally hurting your feelings, speak up. You shouldn't be the butt of *all* the jokes, just because you're pregnant. Sometimes people aren't aware of how self-esteem can be affected during pregnancy. You may have been able to laugh off a few comments about your appearance before, but perhaps you can't handle it now. That's okay. And it's more than okay to say so. You may have to set new boundaries and limits with your friends.

At the same time, start building a support network of mommy friends. If you can't find any, start your own group by hanging a poster in your doctor's waiting room, a local community center, or a baby store. You'll soon learn how important it is to have at least one or two friends with babies around the same age as yours so you can share experiences, ask questions, and trade advice about everything mommy.

But stick by your tried-and-true friends as much as possible even as the pregnancy takes over. Pregnancy is only a temporary phase. Your friends can still be forever.

Husbands, Boyfriends, and Baby Daddies

"Oh yeah, my boys can swim!" That's usually the initial reaction from the man who's fathered your child. Few men can resist the urge to revel in their seminal potency. Sometimes, however, this initial euphoric state wears off quickly. Let's be clear: there are a load of brothers out there who do the Cabbage Patch in excitement for nine months because their queen is with child, and they think their wife has only become sexier with the big boobs and extra pounds. I am not talking about these men—all three of them. I'm talking about the rest of the male population, whom we love and support but understand are somewhat self-centered and have difficulty accepting change. If your man is not as excited, involved, talkative, or obsessive about being prepared for the baby as you are, don't assume the worst. There may be something else afoot. Hold on to something steady, ladies, and hear this: men have deep emotions about pregnancy, too. That may seem hard to believe and even harder to accept when you're lugging a load of groceries and he won't step away from the football game to help you, but it's true. I say this jokingly, but it is a documented fact that most black men

are socialized not to show feelings of anxiety, insecurity, or vulnerability. But these can be very real emotions for any man facing
fatherhood.

Take my husband, for example. I love him dearly, but at times
he has the emotional depth of plywood. But he's a classic male
"fixer"; you know, he wants to fix all problems. And the fact that he
couldn't fix pregnancy—stop the pain, take away my exhausting one
and a half hour commute to New York, end my excruciating back
pain, yadda, yadda, yadda, was too much for him to bear. So as I
complained about my misery and anxieties, he would have a silence
that I mistook for insensitivity and a lack of interest. But he does
not like situations when he does not know what to do. He would
later tell me that he was worried sick about me all the time but
didn't want to show it. What's worse, these nine months would only
culminate with what he couldn't take even more—watching me in
intense pain and with no ability to stop it.

After talking to a few fathers, I found out this wasn't the only
fear in the patch. One of the biggies was financial. These days a lot
of black women are the primary breadwinner or earn just as much
as their husband—either way, the woman's financial contribution is
necessary. Though most of them had a plan for when their wife
would stop and return to work, there were always the "what if"
fears. What if something went wrong and she had to stop working
much earlier than we planned? What if something went wrong and
she couldn't return to work as soon as we need her to? "Just the
thought of not being able to provide for my family properly scared
me, and I knew I couldn't swing it financially on my own," says
James, from Birmingham, Alabama. In their most morbid night-
mares, they saw their wife dying in childbirth and themselves left
with a newborn. The bottom line was that if something goes wrong
with this baby-making business, they would be stuck holding a big
bag of extra pressure. "I definitely felt a lot of stress," James says.

There's also the fear of a changed relationship. Damon from
Pittsburgh, Pennsylvania, admits that he felt displaced by his wife,
Tamika's, pregnancy. "It was clear that she would have less time for

me, and I know it sounds horrible, but I wasn't really cool with that." Your relationship as you know it—with your spontaneous trips, dinners, and quiet nights in—is effectively over. "We had a good life. We traveled, did things together, and even though I really wanted a family, I didn't know how it would change us," Damon says. As many men do, Damon struggled to find his place in this pregnancy period. Nature has already decided what the woman's role is, and all the focus is on her and the baby, leaving the man sitting on the bench.

Women can fear the change, too. "My husband and I have a great life together. I wondered if this baby would really enhance our lives since we do enjoy each other so," says Tanya, of Ann Arbor, Michigan.

Finally, a lot of men were shocked at what pregnancy did to the cool, calm, and collected woman they knew and loved. Husbands didn't expect this grumpy, tired, vomiting person to be part of the pregnancy package. "All of my boys told me horror stories of the crazy things their wives did or made them do during pregnancy. I could have never imagined their wives acting like that, and then it happened to me," recalls Tony, of Baltimore, Maryland.

I offer this insight only to highlight the fact that pregnancy does bring out a response in men. So if your man is acting a little funky or indifferent, there may be a little more to it. Try to be as reassuring as possible. Keep the lines of communication open. Make time to do things together. Some women said that they wished they spent some of their final months doing more things as a couple instead of being consumed in the baby-prep frenzy. Do the best you can. But if tending to your man's emotional needs is draining you, tiring you, and stressing you out, JUST IGNORE HIM; he'll get over it. Don't worry: other women have done this for years. Your focus is the baby.

Another mistake is trying to get your man to understand and empathize with all that you are feeling and experiencing during pregnancy. It will never happen. Classic example: He doesn't read any of the five pregnancy books you left on his nightstand. He's thinking, I've got nine months, that's plenty of time. I'll get to it later. And you think, he doesn't care about me, or this baby, and is completely uninterested in this pregnancy. Or you want him to know how difficult pregnancy is for you, he's thinking how tough it is for him to deal with you, and you'll never agree on who's got it worse. This can typically cause a communication breakdown during pregnancy. Usually it improves after the baby is born, when the "you against me" is replaced by two people in a collaborative effort to keep a freshly baked human alive.

There's another common problem with husbands in pregnancy. All of a sudden, he decides to lose weight and bulk up like LL Cool J, while you're getting fatter by the minute. It happened to Rajine, of Fort Lauderdale, Florida. "Boyfriend was at the gym, dieting, making his muscle building shakes, and I'm sprawled across the couch with my face in a tub of Bon Bons," she says. "I felt like a whale." This is cruel and inhumane treatment and completely unacceptable. If your husband decides to run a marathon, hit the gym, or otherwise drastically improve the look of his body, he is in serious breach of the pregnancy contract. Section V, paragraph 2, clearly states that when a woman is pregnant, all other household members shall remain fat or in their current physical condition. Just tell him to go to the kitchen, make you both an ice cream sundae, and cut out all this crazy talk.

RELATIONSHIP STRESS

Pregnancy can occur at the absolutely, perfectly wrong time. A relationship or marriage may be new or strained. Perhaps you two are more career-focused and never figured children into the picture. I met several women who, with their partner, decided to go off the pill but didn't expect to get pregnant so quickly. There are many who married because a baby was on the way and others who had an unplanned pregnancy in an unhappy relationship. Truth is, there are a lot of babies brought into this world, in spite of, rather than because of, what their parents feel toward each other.

If things aren't so great in your relationship, the months of pregnancy can be used as a time to work together in preparation for the birth. Sandra and her husband, Eddie, from Neptune, New Jersey, were seriously considering divorce when she became pregnant. They didn't know what to do. For the sake of the child, they felt they would try again and if nothing else, work to bring a healthy child into the world. They found a local prenatal group in which couples discussed the effects of pregnancy on their relationship. With therapy, they were able to see things differently and become more sensitive to and understanding of each other's needs. Turns out, they were both just really selfish and wrapped up in what they weren't getting (their words, not mine). But with a baby, you are forced to focus on someone else.

Whatever your relationship with the father of your child may be, he is now a permanent fixture in your life. You may have a good marriage, not-so-good marriage, short-term boyfriend, one-night stand, or, as my girlfriend calls her child's father, "the sperm donor." Knowing that you two can never part ways without having serious complications and adversely affecting the life of a child may bring on anxiety or a sense of security. If this pregnancy was unplanned and you're going through a tough time in your marriage/relationship, you two may want to seek counseling (see Appendix), for the sake of the life you are both bringing into the world, if nothing else.

MOCHA MIX: WHAT THE SISTERS SAY . . .
ABOUT GIRLFRIENDS AND PARTNERS

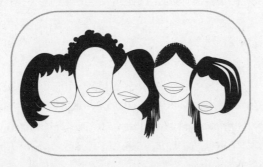

My girlfriends were still my friends but I couldn't share with them all the things I was feeling. They didn't understand what I was going through. Now I was seeking women with similar experiences. My contact with old friends fizzled out. We would speak once a month, or every week. Then it just became few and far between. I needed to be around other mothers. —KUAE, MONTCLAIR, NEW JERSEY

I was the only one who had a child out of all of my girlfriends. And I couldn't go out with them all the time. When your girlfriends don't have kids, they write you off. It's a slow write-off. Is it a written rule somewhere that they call you only so many times and if you turn them down enough they stop calling? I don't know what that number is, but I'm pretty sure that's what happened. Maybe they felt I was pulling away but I was just tired. We never talked about it. It just slowly happened. Even after my first baby, I had separation issues and I didn't want to leave her. That seemed to irritate them. They were like "What's the big deal? Why can't you leave her at home with your husband?" —PHYLLIS, CHICAGO, ILLINOIS

I have truly been blessed by my girls. They took such good care of me. I was spoiled by my friends and everything. If I think about all the hours I made them stroll through the baby superstores with me to look at hundreds of strollers, and still be undecided, it's amazing that they are still my friends. —YVETTE, RICHMOND, VIRGINIA

> *I felt pregnancy brought me and my husband closer together. It was like we were totally united in this shared goal of bringing a new life into the world.*
> —COLLEEN, LONDON, ENGLAND

SPOTLIGHT ON . . .

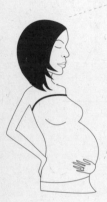

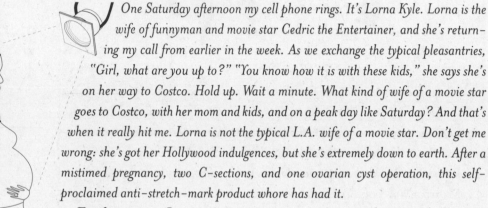

One Saturday afternoon my cell phone rings. It's Lorna Kyle. Lorna is the wife of funnyman and movie star Cedric the Entertainer, and she's return- ing my call from earlier in the week. As we exchange the typical pleasantries, "Girl, what are you up to?" "You know how it is with these kids," she says she's on her way to Costco. Hold up. Wait a minute. What kind of wife of a movie star goes to Costco, with her mom and kids, and on a peak day like Saturday? And that's when it really hit me. Lorna is not the typical L.A. wife of a movie star. Don't get me wrong: she's got her Hollywood indulgences, but she's extremely down to earth. After a mistimed pregnancy, two C-sections, and one ovarian cyst operation, this self- proclaimed anti-stretch-mark product whore has had it.

Finding out I was pregnant was, in a word, overwhelming. Cedric and I were only married two months, and this was not the plan. I wanted to enjoy marriage. I wanted to get it down pat, you know, get it right. Instead here was something that I didn't get to fully embrace, and at the same time I've got this new thing going on. We wanted to travel abroad, and get pregnant when we came back. This wasn't the plan and I was a little disappointed. After I spoke to my husband I snapped out of it. He was so loving and sup- portive. He has that power over me to say one simple thing that changes my feelings and gives me all the security I need. He told me this was a blessing. He said, "God gave us a blessing." And I embraced it from that moment on.

From there on in, I tried to maintain my usual athletic lifestyle. I'm really a big workout person. I grew up in a very athletic house- hold and I was trained to be a world-class runner. I never pursued it, but that conditioning and training have always stuck with me. They cleanse me. I worked out with my trainer and did Pilates for both of my pregnancies. When my trainer was out of town, I did twenty-four laps a day in the pool—it was the only thing I could do by myself without sweating out my hair. With my first, my son Croix, I also did a lot of hiking on the trails of the canyons in L.A.

Cedric would say I had a serious drinking problem, meaning I was thirsty a lot and could down a large amount of liquid before he could blink. Besides that, I do pregnancy really well. People say they want to have a "Lorna Pregnancy." As a professional costumer by trade, everything with me is a production—even pregnancy. And I'm a planner. For instance, I began using plastic sheets on my bed weeks before my due date just in case my water broke while I was sleeping. But I just love the feeling of being encompassed by birth, life, and love. It's the most incredible thing you can do. It's also scary because you don't know what you will be like afterward. I've had my body to myself all those years. I know it well, but it was strange not to know what my body would be like when it was all over.

Delivery and beyond is a different story for me. With my son, I was in labor for twenty-seven hours, but I didn't fully dilate. They gave me some Pitocin but it did not agree with the baby and I had to have an emergency C-section. I was a little disappointed. My baby was fine, but they noticed I had a cyst on my ovary. They watched it for six months and on the seventh month after I had my son, they went back in to clean the ovary. I had a patient female doctor who saw the beauty in keeping it and cared enough to pull the layers back and preserve it. That was important to me because I didn't have a problem getting pregnant again. But it was tough because basically I had two C-sections in one year.

With my second child, I wanted to attempt a vaginal birth, but I was concerned about the risk of a ruptured uterus. I don't like C-sections, but at least I've done that before. I've never pushed anything out. So I said, "I like my uterus. It's been good to me. I don't want to risk it. Let me stick with what I know." I planned my C-section for the same birthday as my sister's. She and my grandfather shared a birthday, but he passed away during my pregnancy so I wanted to do that for her.

That went well, but again, I always get it afterward. After my daughter, Lucky, I was working out really hard to lose the weight, but I had this puffy area around my navel that just wouldn't go down. After about six months, Cedric says something about it. So now I have to go to a doctor because you know when your man comments, you have to do something. The doctor said I had two hernias. I eventually found a reconstructive surgeon who did the procedure through my C-section incision so I didn't have to have another scar. That was another postbaby drama.

During pregnancy I obsessed about two things: avoiding stretch marks and my baby's body parts. First of all, I am a product whore. I can't get enough of them. When I was pregnant I bought everything on the market, from expensive creams to pure glycerin, and I whipped up my own recipes too. At night, I prayed constantly for fingers, nail beds, a pancreas, and a nervous system. Please, God, let my baby have good veins. It kept me up at night.

Now I tell women try not to worry, because it always works out. When you worry you put that stress on your baby and you don't want that.

ReTell Therapy

FROM FAB TO FLAB: MY PREGNANCY JOURNEY

by Jennifer Mischel-Wilson

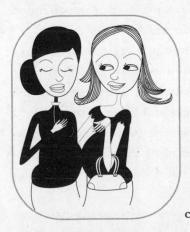

My husband and I didn't even want kids. For me, it wasn't that I don't love children, but I felt like I had done it all already. As the oldest of four children, I have always had a big role in my siblings' life, and that of my nieces and nephews. Before I married I found myself playing mommy to about a total of seven kids. It was a crazy life.

While I'm happily working on marriage and pursuing my career goals—I wanted to become district manager for the retail company I work for—my sister drops a bombshell: she's having a baby and she needed my help. This was hard to digest because my sister was in her third year in college, single, and we have very strict old-fashioned Haitian parents who do not approve of premarital sex or unwed mothers. What's more, just when I thought I was free of helping with someone else's kids, it was like, here we go again.

I had to figure out how to support my sister, be a good wife, and continue to perform at a stressful job. My sister's pregnancy only reaffirmed what I already knew. "I know for sure I'm not having a baby," I told my husband.

As my sister approached her due date, two of my bosses met with me and said that I was finally going to be promoted. I was proud and pleased. I only asked for one month before accepting the position because I was my sister's birth partner and her due date was near. The big day for the birth of my nephew finally arrives. During delivery I saw things no woman needs to see or they will not, I mean, *not*, have a baby. I never knew that a little vagina could look so ugly, and get so big, and endure so much pain. After all that, I said to my hubby once again with all my conviction—"There is no way I'm ever, ever having a baby."

On the way home we stopped at a drugstore and I saw a sale on a home pregnancy test. I figured it might be good to have one in the house. As I got ready for bed, my curiosity got the best of me. I said, "Let's see how accurate these so-called tests are." I took it with no fear. In less than ten seconds I saw two bright lines. I couldn't believe it. My sister delivers and I find out I'm pregnant on the same day! It couldn't be! I took four more pregnancy tests and saw two different doctors before I allowed myself to accept the news.

First, I had to tell my job I couldn't take the position. I was crushed, because I worked so hard to get what I really wanted. But I had to make a choice: Who comes first? The baby or me? From that day on, I became a mom.

One day, when I was only three and a half months along, I had some excruciating pain and I went to the emergency room. They told me that I had placenta previa—a very serious condition. Placenta previa means that the placenta is before the baby and the baby is lying on top of it. You feel pain and pressure and have frequent spotting. If the placenta doesn't reverse, you must deliver by C-section, because if you go into labor and the baby starts to push on the placenta you can hemorrhage.

This really upset me because I had told my own doctor several times about the pain I was having but she told me, "Don't worry; it's just your uterus growing." She never checked it out. She gave me no personal attention and she never remembered my name. After that I quickly switched doctors, and I tell all women never to stick with a physician who doesn't take a personal interest in you and your pregnancy.

After a four-month bout with morning sickness, or in my case, all-day sickness, I really hit my pregnancy stride. My skin was glowing, my nails were growing, and my hair was flowing. I must say, I looked good. But I had no sex drive—this is so not my style. My poor husband was going crazy! I would try to get in the mood, but seeing him naked made me nauseous. Sex seemed like hard work as my body got bigger and bigger.

By the time I was eight and a half months the doctor told me two things. First, the placenta had reversed itself. I was so happy I started to cry. Second, she warned me about my weight gain. My prepregnancy weight was about one hundred thirty pounds. But I was constantly hungry, so I constantly ate. I was now about two hundred pounds and would top two hundred twenty pounds before delivery.

My labor wasn't so bad, but afterward was hard. I couldn't believe that I was pregnant for ten long months and in just a few hours it was all over. I had a little person in my arms that was my very own. I challenge anyone to give birth and then say there is no God. Adjusting to motherhood and losing weight became my next journey.

My best advice is to go easy on the pregnancy TV shows. They can make you very nervous. And don't listen to anyone's horror story, either. Everyone has her own experience. Just take care of yourself on the inside and out. Get your hair and nails done; put on some nice clothes and a little bit of makeup. Having a baby is the most beautiful and rewarding thing you will ever do in your life. So pamper yourself and let everyone else pamper you, also. Honey, after those nine months are over, you won't get any attention.

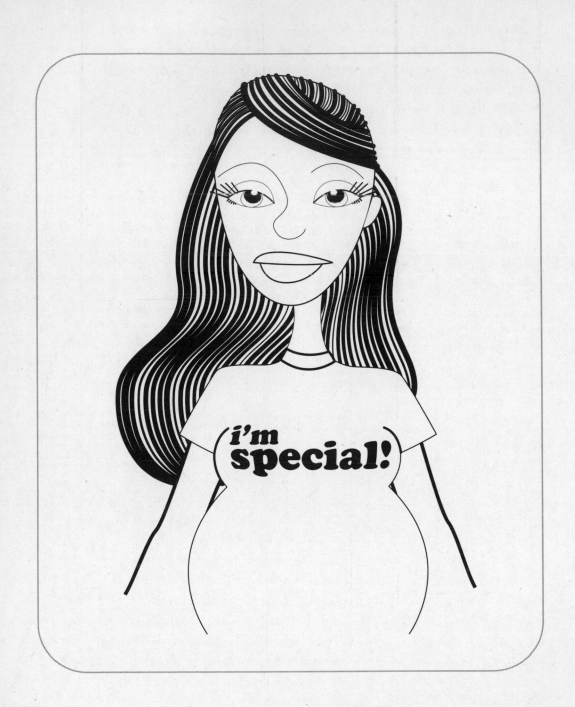

5

Not Your Ordinary Pregnancy

SINGLE MOTHER, HAVING TWINS, OVER AGE THIRTY-FIVE

It's not easy to be pregnant on your own, but it does happen. Even to those to whom society says these things should never happen. But it does. Although happily married now, my husband and I were unwed when my oldest daughter was conceived while I was working in London. He's British. The shock of an unplanned pregnancy was more than our relatively new relationship could handle. He decided to stay in Britain and I returned to the States. Months into the pregnancy, he severed ties completely. It was the most difficult time in my life. Feelings of abandonment, shame, and loneliness cloaked me like a heavy blanket. A year later, he reconnected with our child and later with me. We reestablished our spiritual base, worked through our feelings in therapy, and learned the true meaning of forgiveness. Still, it is just not one of those things you will ever get over; it's something you just continually work through.

So I fully understand that birth control fails, relationships fall apart, divorce and separation happen, or people die—and that any one of these situations can leave a woman pregnant in circumstances that she least expected. And these women are not always the stereotypical teenager, or uneducated woman, or poor woman. They may be college educated or have well-paying jobs, some double-degreed, with a solid career, and in their midtwenties, thirties, and beyond.

No matter how you got into the situation, when you are alone and pregnant, the typical congratulatory comments and all the best wishes and excitement about pregnancy may not be coming your way as readily. Instead, news of your pregnancy may bring on inappropriate comments of disapproval or insensitive remarks about your decision to carry this baby. It can be an emotionally trying time for even the strongest of women.

Being a single mother has its own additional stressors. I never noticed that nearly every woman in every advertisement or photo in a pregnancy magazine is wearing a wedding band until I didn't have one on my finger. It made me sad, depressed, and resentful even to see the subtle ways that society views unwed moms-to-be. Then there are the challenges of awkward glances from strangers, financial worries, or painful conflicts with your family or the father of your child. I found myself just fraught with anxiety, even about things that were years down the road, like paying for college or, if I had a boy, how I would teach him to pee standing up. All of these anxieties, both the immediate ones and the simply neurotic ones, can be emotionally taxing at a time when raging hormones and the physical demands of pregnancy are already more than enough to deal with.

The initial shock of accepting this pregnancy and then telling others is often the hardest part. But it will wear off. "Put your tough skin on," as my great-grandmother says. Don't let anyone make you feel bad or foolish because of your decision—no one has that right. Your baby is just as precious as one conceived through a marital bond, and a child can be successfully raised by a single parent these days.

But no matter what anybody tells you, or how self-reliant and confident you are, facing disapproval from loved ones is tough. Facing disapproval from strangers isn't easy, either. I distinctly recall sitting on a bus riding across 125th Street in Harlem with my ringless hands clasped over my bump. An elderly black woman boarded, with her shiny black pocketbook and print scarf tied neatly under her neck. Being a respectful girl with southern roots I gave a cordial smile when our eyes crossed. But my smile was not returned; instead she just stared at my belly with a disapproving menace. At first I thought my own hypersensitivity about the situation was making me feel that all old black ladies were staring at me with disdain, but it happened over and over again. I wanted to write a sign on my forehead that read: *I am not another teenage pregnancy statistic. I am twenty-nine and I have a master's degree from Columbia University, damn it!* But it didn't matter. From then on, I found myself avoiding eye contact with certain black people. I felt horrible! But sadly, many single women said that they received the most unkind treatment from other black folks, particularly women.

One woman, a Yale graduate, was in a loving, committed relationship—but unmarried—when she became pregnant. She tells of the unsympathetic treatment she received at her predominantly black female workplace. "There was this, 'Well, you got yourself into this situation, so you deal with it like I dealt with it' kind of attitude," she says.

Being alone and pregnant made me really miss my Granny. My great-grandmother and I had a great relationship, and in the long summers I spent roasting like a pig in the South Carolina heat, we bonded in ways that made other relatives jealous. To Granny, I could do no wrong, until I actually did wrong and she would lovingly let me have it. But my Granny was my original cheerleader. Before I realized how crucial it is for a black woman in this society to have a cheering squad, my Granny was mine. I just knew that if somehow she were still alive, she would be able to say just the right thing to assure me that I could make it through this pregnancy. Instead, I pored through shoe boxes of old photos of Granny and me, reveling in the happy memories, remembering the things she told me, and feeling strengthened by her unwavering confidence in my abilities. Everyone needs a Granny or her own cheering squad to get through a pregnancy alone. Establish your own circle of support—which may or may not be family members. Sometimes the family we create for ourselves is stronger than the one we were born in. Your goal is to find the friends who will listen and respond positively—not lecture or judge you. By identifying even one ally, you will have someone to turn to when others react negatively. Simone, a thirty-two-year-old office manager from New York, was shocked when her parents refused to help her out during her pregnancy. But she had one sister who helped her financially and encouraged her to stay positive. Brianna, from Washington, D.C., wrote letters to her unborn child as a way of connecting to him, and as an outlet for her conflicting emotions.

Another offense against negative people is a good defense. I often found myself so thrown off by the rude comments that I didn't know what to say; I kind of just stood there with a Ralph Kramden, Homm-mina Homm-mina Homm-mina thing going on. Try to be prepared for the possible criticisms and have a response. For example, if someone says, "You're ruining your future," you can say something like "My life won't stop because I have a child. I may have to put a few things off for a little while, but the joys of being with my child will be more than worth it." Or if someone says, "A child needs a father," say, "I know. And I will do everything possible to make sure the father or a number of suitable role models are around for him/her." Also, show how committed you are to doing this single mother thing right. Mention that you're reading parenting books, taking a particular parenting class, researching on the Web, or joining a support group or other organization. Not only will you be talking a good game, but you'll be further convincing yourself that you *can* do this.

If friends and relatives aren't a support option for you, find local pregnancy support groups by looking in the yellow pages, searching the Internet, checking local bulletin boards in your area, or contacting the National Black Women's Health Project (see Appendix), which has self-help groups for single mothers across the country.

If these avenues don't work or you find that dealing with your pregnancy, your parents' disapproval, the father's anger or attitude, and your own worries about handling the future has you feeling on the brink of an emotional collapse, please get yourself some professional help. Do not be afraid of a little couch time. Sometimes getting counseling from an unbiased, trained professional can help you keep your sanity. Once you've got yourself centered and feeling strong again, it's time to start thinking about the other person who helped create this life—the father. Consider what is best for your child, trying to put aside any bitterness or anger you may feel toward the father. The truth of the matter is, it's very difficult for most women, even with a sizable paycheck, to raise a child with no contribution whatsoever from the other parent. Everybody knows someone who has done it, but everyone will also tell you how incredibly difficult it was. Begin thinking about ways that the two of you can share responsibility for this child, including financial support, child care and school costs, custody and visitation, emotional involvement, family participation, life insurance for the father with the child as a beneficiary, life insurance for the child, armed forces benefits, health insurance, savings toward college, and even inheritance. You may hate your boyfriend now or you may love him now and hate him later, but focus on what's in the best interest of the child. A special word of caution here: Sometimes our girlfriends are looking out for us, or think they are looking out for us, with a lot of the "You don't need that loser" or "Forget him; you got us" kind of talk. Now if they are trying to help you stay out of a bad relationship, that's one thing, but if they are talking about cutting the child off from her father, that's another matter. True, you may not need him (though I would argue that on some levels you do), but that child most definitely does need her father!

Stay focused on your baby. Think of several options for contributing or coparenting and write them down. Get your Johnny Cochran on, and start researching the law. If you don't know what type of support to expect, find your state's Child Support Enforcement office, county courthouse, or librarian to help you find your state's guidelines as defined by its Family Law Code. Draft a document that includes an acknowledgment of paternity, the amount of money given for support, the identity of the custodial parent, when and how long visitations will be, how much life insurance the father should have for the child, and the like. Discuss it and negotiate with the father, keeping the focus on the child, rather than on either of you. Have the document checked by an attorney to make sure it complies with the laws of your state, and then sign it, get it notarized, and even have it filed with the courts before your third trimester. First of all, babies come early. Second, with all the anxiety of impending childbirth, the last thing you want to worry about is whether this man is going to pull a fast one on you or flip the script after the birth. Taking the legal approach shows the father you are serious about parenting and about his living up to his legal responsibility. Many women never actually had to use these documents but could rest easy knowing they were in place. As one very sassy, Joan Clayton—like family attorney once told me, "Every unmarried pregnant woman should be seeing a doctor *and* a lawyer."

I would also toss in a financial planner. Babies can wreak havoc on a two-income household, not to mention a one-paycheck home. But just because you're a single mother doesn't mean you'll be relegated to a life of eating Ramen noodles or tuna fish every night. It does mean starting early to get a budget in place, practicing a little discipline, and saving like your life depended on it. See Chapter Twelve to get your financial house in order.

Twins

Did you know that African Americans have the highest rates of twins? In fact, the Yoruba Oshogbo tribe in Nigeria has the world's highest rates of twin births. That means you have a higher chance of conceiving twins just because you're black. The rates are sixteen out of every one thousand births for blacks, eight out of every one thousand births for whites, and four or fewer out of every one thosand births for Asians. For fraternal twins only, the rates jump to 28.8 per one thousand births for blacks, versus 19.6 per one thousand births for whites. If you're reading this section, I'm assuming that you have been so blessed. Congratulations! Talk about a fertility mama! Remember those TV shows or movies in which an unsuspecting mother delivers a baby, and just as she recovers with a smile, there's the shocking news that there's another baby on the way out? Thanks to sonograms, all those blood tests, and the monitors that can pick up more than one fetal heartbeat, those things rarely happen anymore. Now that I think about it, strangely, it did happen in the series finale of *Friends*—but that show was never anything like real life anyway!

I can rattle on for hours about my fascination with twin births—the connection between fraternal twins, who share the same intrauterine environment for seven to nine months, the whole sensing of each other forever—it's really amazing. When I get started on one of these rants with mothers of twins about all the metaphysical aspects of twins, they quickly yank me off that trip with a reality check: double strollers, two feedings, two babies crying at the same time, two babies to toilet-train, and yet a woman who still only has two hands. It's not as if giving birth to twins means you sprout extra limbs, or your health insurance gives you a baby nurse to help with the extra load. You'll be dealing with all of that soon enough.

Right now, you may still be trying to come to grips with the initial shock of carrying twins. If the anxiety of becoming a mother of one child is taxing, the mere thought of dealing with the demands of two babies can be overwhelming and downright scary. All of your ideas of what childbirth and the adjustment period afterward may be like are thrown out the window now that you're expecting twins. "My husband and I were petrified. We faked excitement to others, but we were scared stiff," says Keishawn, a physical therapist in Los Angeles. If you're ambivalent about your double-trouble pregnancy, don't beat yourself up with guilt. Plenty of women have felt similarly. Talk to your partner, or find a parents of twins support group, or, at the very least, the name of a mother of twins in your area, to get some advice. On the other hand, there are plenty of women who are over the moon about twins. Some of them wanted more than one child anyway, and the thought of getting a twofer, that is, two kids with only one pregnancy, was like hitting Lotto!

Of course, a twin pregnancy is more stressful and physically demanding. Because your double load has to share the space in the uterus and the nutrients that sometimes pass through only one placenta, twins often have low birth weight—though I recently met a woman who gave birth to two eight-pound twins. God bless her! Her husband should have shown up with diamonds after that feat. Still, a multiple pregnancy is considered high risk, so you'll have a strict schedule of office visits and endless tests. Since a preterm birth is a major complication of multiple pregnancies, your doctor will be checking your cervix, often as early as twenty weeks, to detect any signs of premature dilatation. There's also a greater chance of your activities being restricted and of being put on bed rest or hospitalized, which can be frustrating for women who are typically quite active. The good news is that carrying twins makes you the person who can legitimately claim to eat for two during pregnancy—you'll need an additional three hundred calories a day on top of the recommended pregnancy caloric intake, along with an extra protein serving, one extra calcium serving, and an extra whole grain serving. In fact, carrying twins means even more careful attention to your diet. Doctors say that proper nutrition is the best way to combat the common low-birth-weight problem of multiple pregnancies. You absolutely cannot skimp on protein, vitamins, and minerals. Protein is the building block of every cell in your body and in your babies' bodies. It will help you build a good placenta and a strong amniotic sac. A healthy diet will also help fight against infection. Twins fed by a better diet can weigh in at a healthier six to seven pounds or more. Sounds good, until you factor in the supersized morning sickness, doubled intestinal discomforts, and a stomach that's being squeezed sooner by a stuffed uterus. Tamia of Greensboro, North Carolina, says she felt full all the time and just couldn't get any more food in. She found that cutting out the stuff she wanted, but that didn't have much nutritional value, helped save room for the good stuff. She also ate about six times a day plus snacks, rather than going for three meals a day. If possible, get some help with preparing nutritious meals, and you may also need a hand with housework during pregnancy.

Extra iron may also be necessary during pregnancy, as maternal anemia is a common problem in multiple pregnancies, but try to eat iron-rich foods rather than taking an iron supplement, which can lead to constipation—you don't need any more drama. Drink lots of water, too; shoot for a minimum of two quarts a day, since the risk of premature contractions and early delivery increases if you become dehydrated. Your doctor may make other recommendations.

There are other common problems of twin pregnancies:

* Preeclampsia, or pregnancy-induced high blood pressure, develops in about 10 to 20 percent of women carrying twins, twice the rate of women pregnant with one baby.
* Placental abruption, in which the placenta detaches from the uterine wall before delivery, is more common when you're carrying twins. But most studies have linked the problem to malnutrition and smoking, and I know those don't apply to anyone reading this book. It is rare among well-nourished women.
* Fetal growth restriction occurs when one or both twins aren't growing at the proper rate. This may cause the babies to be

born prematurely or at a low birth weight. Almost half of pregnancies with more than one baby have this problem.

✳ Twin-to-twin transfusion syndrome occurs when one twin takes the other's blood supply. This is a rare but serious complication in identical twins: one baby is getting too much blood and the other too little. As serious as this condition is, survival rates these days are much higher because of early detection.

Thanks to the advancements of medical science, today's moms have great outcomes from twin births. More than 90 percent of twin births go off without a hitch. So don't listen to all the scary stories about multiple pregnancies; focus on the positive ones. For multiple pregnancies, thirty-six weeks is your magic number. Once you get to about thirty-six weeks, you're considered out of the danger zone, and the risk of delivering a premature or low-birth-weight baby drops considerably.

Mothers of twins tell me constantly that twins start taking their toll from the very beginning. Soledad O'Brien, CNN *American Morning* anchor, had fraternal twin boys and two daughters in the span of four years. With her first two pregnancies she, in her own words, "worked till the end and popped them out—no problem." The twins were a completely different story (read more from Soledad on page 136). Morning sickness was more severe, back pain was more severe, and dehydration was a problem. Remember all the things you read about in Chapter One: the slowing digestive system, the aches and pains, and the morning sickness. Well, multiply that by two. Or, as some women tell it, by ten. There is extra pressure on your digestive system and on your diaphragm and lungs not to mention the extra stress on your spine and other bones. Varicose veins, shortness of breath, and constipation can also wreak double havoc. Your muscles take a brutal beat down as well, because your stomach, pelvic floor, legs, feet, shoulders, arms, and back all have to support the extra weight and still get you through your normal daily routine. One of the best remedies, and I use that word loosely because there is only so much relief possible, is getting more rest. Your body is working twice as hard as it would with a single pregnancy and is being doubly sapped of all the good stuff. Rest helps you better deal with all the physical demands of carrying twins and gives your body a little time to recover. It can also help with the crankiness and frustration of carrying such a load. Rest, however, does not necessarily mean sleep. It does mean doing as many things as you can sitting comfortably with your feet up. To make yourself more comfortable, get some real support for your back in the form of cushions, foam wedges, or masses of pillows, which can help make the exaggerated curve of the lower spine a little more comfortable.

With the extra baby comes the extra weight gain: not just the fat from all the ice cream you're craving, but all that extra baby stuff—an extra placenta and amniotic fluid. You're expected to gain thirty-five to forty-five pounds, about ten pounds more than the charts say for women with single pregnancies. On the other hand, you need to gain enough weight so your babies can grow to a healthy size. Talk to your doctor, since your personal recommended weight gain will be related to your prepregnancy weight.

Today, twin births don't have to be delivered by C-section. Vaginal births are considered safe and are encouraged. In fact, doctors know that the stimulation and rise in hormone levels that come with labor actually benefit the babies. Still, twin births almost always necessitate delivering in the hospital. So if you were envisioning a cozy home birth with candles and a little Luther playing in the background, you may be disappointed. Whether or not you will have a vaginal birth will depend on many factors, including the position of the babies and how well the babies tolerate labor.

Over Age Thirty-five

More and more women are having babies later in life. With women pursuing higher education, launching a career, and waiting for Mr. Right, making babies gets pushed further along. All the while a woman is juggling the options. "Do I have babies early on when there are less pregnancy risks and I have more energy to chase a toddler? Or do I wait until I have more job security (so I can afford to take a maternity leave without losing my job) and a bigger paycheck, even though I may have more difficulty getting pregnant or there may be other health dangers?" Before you know it, you turn around and you're thirty years old, with a boom-banging career and no marriage prospects in sight. Others marry in their early thirties and spend a few years solidifying their marriage relationship and preparing financially before starting a family. Then there's the perennial "waiting for the right time" group. And don't forget about the sisters on a second marriage or, better yet, a second marriage to a much younger man (yummy!) who want to have a child with their new mate. Whatever the reasons, it is certainly happening. According to data compiled by the government, black women above age thirty-five and into their forties are having more pregnancies, even while the rate among the twenty-something women declines.

This is a marked change of course for black folks. Perhaps your mother or grandmother married in her late teens, or as early as sixteen in some cases in the South. Back then, women were finished childbearing in their thirties, which was considered more like middle age than it is now. Times are different. I met plenty of black women who had their first child at forty and then went back for seconds. Wasn't it Miss Diva Diana Ross who had a son at forty-two and then another a year later? Having a baby later in life can provoke insensitive comments and questions from your mama and other older kinfolk. That goes to show that pregnancy is one area that hasn't caught up with modern thinking about age thirty-five. I mean, isn't that the age when we reach our sexual peak, spread our wings, and get our groove back, or was that just Terry McMillan feeding us some bull? Just when we're hitting our stride in terms of being at peace with our career, relationships, and spirituality, the medical lot says we're too old for childbearing. Yet, some of us spent so much time at the office in our twenties and early thirties, we had to leave Post-it note reminders to eat, see a doctor, or have sex with our husband.

That's why I find this magic number of thirty-five pretty hard to deal with. So many black women I met while researching this book were just hitting full throttle as they approached the midthirties. We look great (you know black don't crack!), we feel fabulous, and we have a little sassy bounce in our step that only comes from feeling good from within and knowing you got it goin' on. Stacey, a leggy sister from New York, had her first child at thirty-five and felt she was in some frantic race against the clock to get a child in before thirty-four. "The pressure, even from my own doctor, was unbelievable," she says. I also spoke to childless older women who may have had perfectly uncomplicated pregnancies but were scared off by all the doom and gloom about post-thirty-five pregnancies. "It seemed like it was now or never at thirty-five. But it really wasn't and I wished we had tried anyway," says Sandra, forty-eight, of Birmingham, Alabama. For those who find themselves wanting children, witnessing the media's fear campaign about declining fertility and increasing risks can bring on a lot of anguish.

Not that there aren't more concerns with being pregnant over age thirty-five. If you scour the Internet, you'll be frightened to pieces by all the risk words out there, *placenta previa, preeclampsia,* and the *prolapse* of a number of things. Not that you won't need special care, but please don't let anyone make you feel like a prehistoric relic. Nor should you be scared to death. Really, the problem is not you—you're healthy, vivacious, and fierce—it's your eggs. You see, a woman is born with all the eggs she will ever have. So at forty, you've got forty-year-old eggs; meanwhile boyfriend is pumping out a batch of fresh sperm all the time. The longer an egg sits around in the ovaries, the more likely it is to develop a chromosomal abnormality. Sperm only takes about ninety days to mature. So getting pregnant at thirty-five requires the meeting of ninety-day-old sperm with thirty-five-year-old eggs.

That union doesn't occur without risks. One is that a preexisting medical condition can be more pronounced. That means if you have high blood pressure, fibroids, or diabetes prior to conception, they are more likely to cause complications during your pregnancy. There is also a greater chance for the development of gestational diabetes or pregnancy-induced hypertension. Older moms-to-be also have a higher risk of a miscarriage. For younger women, the chance of a miscarriage is about 15 percent, or one in eight pregnancies that ends in miscarriage. At age thirty-five the rate rises to one in four, and at forty the miscarriage rate is nearly one in three. The risk of an emergency C-section also rises to about 15 percent in this age group.

Women over thirty-five also have a higher risk of postlabor stress incontinence—a strange way of saying unexpected urine leakage when laughing, coughing, or sneezing. Doing the Kegels—squeezing the same set of muscles you would use to stop your urine midstream—to strengthen your pelvic floor can help. Tighten and hold for a count of 10, and then release for a count of 10, and repeat. Do this ten times, about three times a day.

One of the worst anxieties is the increased chance of a birth defect. Babies born to older mothers are more likely to have conditions caused by abnormal chromosomes, the most common of which is Down's syndrome. Despite many years of research to identify the risk factors of Down's syndrome, only maternal age has been well established, according to the Centers for Disease Control. The risk of having a baby who has Down's syndrome begins to increase at age thirty-five and slowly rises with age. Family history and cigarette smoking while using oral contraceptives have also been shown to increase the risk in a few studies. At age thirty-five, the chance of Down's syndrome is slightly less than 0.5 percent. That means that more than 99 percent of pregnancies at that age will not have the abnormality. The risk rises to 3 percent by age forty-five, which is still 97 percent without Down's syndrome. Either way, all women in the United States who will deliver at age thirty-five are offered a number of tests. The most common is amniocentesis.

Amniocentesis is a procedure that removes some amniotic fluid from around the baby. With ultrasound guidance, a long needle is inserted through your abdomen and into the amniotic sac. That fluid contains many fetal cells, which can be analyzed in a lab for any abnormalities. It is usually done in the second trimester at about sixteen weeks. Another option for a couple in the high-risk group—as defined by the doctor—who don't want to wait until week sixteen is to get a chorionic villius sampling or (CVS) test in the first trimester, often as early as eleven weeks. Women who strongly prefer the option to terminate a pregnancy with an abnormality before the first trimester ends should discuss the CVS test with their doctor. Be aware that the CVS test has a slightly higher risk of test-related miscarriage than the amnio. Some studies put the amniocentesis risk at less than one in two hundred, compared to one in one hundred for the CVS. The CVS is performed either with a transcervical tube through the vaginal canal and into the cervix or with a long needle that is inserted into the abdomen and through the uterus. Either way, a tiny piece of the villi—the finger-like projections of tissue that attach the placenta to the wall of the uterus—is extracted. It contains the same genetic makeup as the baby and is checked in a lab for defects.

For days Laura and Jamal, from Dallas, deliberated on whether or not to have genetic testing. She was thirty-seven years old, and Jamal, who never knew his father, had recently learned of a cousin who had Down's syndrome. On the one hand, they felt blessed to have conceived after age thirty-five and a year of trying, and they didn't want to lose the baby because of the test. "But could we handle a child with special needs? I mean, financially and emotionally, is this the family we wanted? The questions kept coming," Laura says. "We must have gone back and forth one hundred times. But in the end we decided what God gives, we take." Their baby boy was, in Laura's words, "perfect." Many sisters who wouldn't terminate the pregnancy regardless of the outcome opted not to have the amnio-centesis. Instead, they relied on their faith and the belief that they would somehow handle whatever their child turned out to be. Others chose to terminate. Ann from Decatur, Georgia, wanted the amniocentesis so she could be prepared. "I didn't plan to terminate, but I felt I wanted to know if I would have a child with special needs." If you do plan to keep the baby regardless of a genetic disorder, you should still consider testing early. Studies show that early intervention and care can improve your child's quality of life.

There are also a few noninvasive options to check for genetic abnormalities. You can choose the noninvasive methods first, then go for a CVS or amnio only if there is a sign of a problem. One such option uses an ultrasound scan at between ten and fourteen weeks to measure the thickness of tissues at the back of the baby's neck (nuchal tissues), sometimes referred to as a measurement of nuchal translucency. In about a third of the cases when they find thick neck skin, the baby is totally normal and healthy. The other two-thirds of the time, however, this thick neck skin is evidence of Down's syndrome or other abnormalities. The ultrasound is considered a "marker," not a definite finding, of Down's syndrome.

Another is the triple-screen or quad-screen blood test. This test can indicate any increased risks for Down's syndrome or spina bifida (a problem that occurs when the spine hasn't fused closed properly, causing the spinal cord and its membranes to protrude out of the infant's back; there is no known cause of spina bifida, but it is related to a deficiency in folic acid—something a prenatal vitamin pill high in folic acid can help prevent). In this screen, the mother's blood is tested for markers in three or four chemistry tests. The results of this test plus the mother's age, mother's weight, and the baby's gestational age are plugged into a computer that pops out a number that assesses the risk level for your pregnancy. A 1:5,000 risk of Down's syndrome would be a very low, minimal risk that wouldn't require further testing, and a 1:10 risk would be considered high, so your doctor would likely recommend an amnio. Even with the high risk level of 1:10, there is still a 90 percent chance that the baby is normal. A spina bifida screen result that indicates a "normal" or "increased" risk level would require further testing.

If you're really concerned, perhaps because of a family history of

Down's syndrome, you can see a genetic counselor, who can factor in the ultrasound, blood screening result, your family history, your age, and other risk factors to give you a personal risk assessment of having a baby who has Down's syndrome. After giving themselves quite a scare, a lot of women were surprised to find out how low their actual risk was.

The good news for the over-thirty-five crew is that research also shows that babies born to older women are breast-fed longer, do better at school, and are more likely to have parents who stay together than babies born to younger women. Older mothers are also statistically happier to become stay-at-home moms, since they may have already fulfilled their career ambitions. And they tend to be more financially stable.

Mocha Mix: What the Sisters Say . . . About Being a Single Mother, Having Twins, and Over Thirty-five

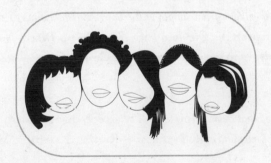

On My Own

I thought I couldn't have children, so when I got pregnant I was so happy—married or not. —Lisa, Buffalo, New York

We were together for eleven years and I never, in a million years, thought we would have problems. He wasn't supportive of the pregnancy and finally after our son was born we broke up. My girlfriends chipped in to cover the costs of getting a lawyer to draw up a custody and child support agreement. I thought it was crazy at the time, because I thought I knew him so well. Years later, he married and started acting, well, stupid, and I was ever so thankful for that legal document. —DIANNE, NEW BRUNSWICK, NEW JERSEY

I was determined to bring my child into a drama-free zone. I started surrounding myself with positive, supportive people and basically cut off everyone else. No one is worth getting stressed out during my pregnancy or creating a negative vibe for my child's birth. —PAM, CHICAGO, ILLINOIS

My girlfriend made me a CD of empowering anthems like "I'm Every Woman," "Survivor," "Ain't No Stoppin Us Now," "Respect," and "I Will Survive," along with a few of those man-hating, I'm-better-off-without-you-type hits. Every time I felt a little down, I would pop it in, sing my heart out, and dance around a little bit. It was my own kind of therapy session. —MAISHA, LOS ANGELES, CALIFORNIA

We decided not to do the shotgun wedding thing—not to mention that the thought of one of those pregnant bridal gowns made me cringe. But we did everything together—from shopping for baby stuff to Lamaze—and he was incredibly supportive. Our love grew from the experience. Now we're a happy family. —SHAVONDA, ATLANTA, GEORGIA

Twins

I was shocked that I was having twins. I've never been so completely excited and scared out of my mind at the same time. —RENEE, LANSING, MICHIGAN

At first my twins seemed to be growing at unequal rates, which freaked me out. In the end, the one growing too slowly outpaced the other twin and their measurements reversed, which was a big relief. In the end, I had two healthy babies. —STEPHANIE, WASHINGTON, D.C.

I had some problems with premature labor. Twice, I was sent to the hospital, given intravenous fluids, monitored, and sent home. But I made it past the thirty-seven weeks stage and brought home my healthy twin boys. —LOUANN, KNOXVILLE, TENNESSEE

I had pretty much a problem-free pregnancy. I delivered my twins vaginally about five minutes apart at thirty-six weeks; it was so amazing.
—DARCELLE, LONDON, ENGLAND

Over Thirty-five

Just when my family was focused on SATs and colleges for my seventeen-year-old, I was pregnant again at forty-two. I was nervous about all the things they say advanced age can mean to a pregnancy, but my labor was the shortest of all my children and I had a smooth delivery. —DONNA, OAKLAND, CALIFORNIA

When I was in my twenties and early thirties I was a mess. I was in no shape to be somebody's mother. Now I feel a lot more emotionally stable and more prepared for motherhood. —CHERITA, GARY, INDIANA

At age thirty-nine—with a twenty- and a seventeen-year-old already—it is like starting all over. People say stupid things like "Oh, you're so brave. I wouldn't do that." One doctor said, "That's what you get for marrying a young buck. Why would you want to go back to bottles?" It's hard not to react or be hurt. I was very afraid that my age would cause problems. I threw myself into work as a distraction. —DEBBIE, LOS ANGELES, CALIFORNIA

SPOTLIGHT ON . . .
SOLEDAD O'BRIEN, A TWIN STORY

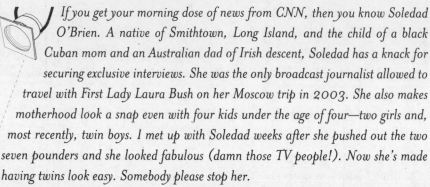

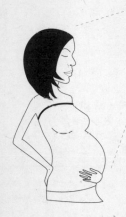

If you get your morning dose of news from CNN, then you know Soledad O'Brien. A native of Smithtown, Long Island, and the child of a black Cuban mom and an Australian dad of Irish descent, Soledad has a knack for securing exclusive interviews. She was the only broadcast journalist allowed to travel with First Lady Laura Bush on her Moscow trip in 2003. She also makes motherhood look a snap even with four kids under the age of four—two girls and, most recently, twin boys. I met up with Soledad weeks after she pushed out the two seven pounders and she looked fabulous (damn those TV people!). Now she's made having twins look easy. Somebody please stop her.

This pregnancy was incredibly difficult from the moment I got pregnant. Everything came early, often, and twice as bad. With my first two, I started feeling a little nauseous around eight weeks, but with the twins I was violently ill at three weeks. I couldn't even keep water down. I was throwing up five times a day. It was awful. At work, on the set, my coanchor would cover for me. I'm thankful I could control the vomiting. So I could vomit, clean up, get my hair fixed, and be back in action in about four minutes. I tried everybody's tricks—ginger, crackers—nothing worked. I tried small meals, but then I would just have a big fat meal since I would throw it up in twenty-five minutes anyway. And it didn't stop there. My two girls would bring home these twenty-four-hour bugs, I would get the virus, and because I couldn't hold anything down, I ended up dehydrated and hospitalized. Dehydration can lead to contractions, which can lead to preterm labor. A couple of times, I was starting to go into preterm labor, but there wasn't anything medically wrong with me.

That's the thing about pregnancy. Babies take everything from you until you have nothing left to give and then it's time to come out. During the course of thirty-eight weeks I developed sciatica, somehow ripped the muscles in my rib cage, and later I developed some viral thing that builds up under your skin or something, so I was chronically itching.

Funny enough, medically speaking, it was a great, healthy pregnancy. But I was just wiped out all of the time. In the end, I was put on bed rest eight weeks early. Intellectually, I knew it was a very smart thing to be on bed rest, but it was very hard for me not to work. I was healthy before I became pregnant. I thought it would be a breeze. I worked to the bitter end with my other two, but I realized that you can have two healthy babies or you can work yourself to death. Still, I felt annoyed with myself because I had to stop work. I was trying to get everything done, and I dropped some of the balls. Lots of professional women are used to juggling a lot of things and then pregnancy comes and we don't really think of it as a deviation from our lives. My doctor told me, you can either put the time in for a healthy pregnancy and healthy baby or not take care of yourself and end up spending all your time after delivery in the intensive care unit nursing your sick babies to health. Either way, you will put in the time, he says. I'm just glad I didn't have a C-section. I didn't have time for the longer recovery of a C-section.

I had an epidural. They usually do that with twins. I struggled every step of the way to push those boys out and I'm proud of it. There's such a high C-section rate with twins. My boys were big babies, and I love big babies, and delivery was surprisingly fast.

After four children, I don't worry about my body image. My body is what it is. And I have stretch marks on top of stretch marks. I'm just a passenger on this train.

A lot of viewers write in saying that I'm a supermom, and asking, "How do you do it?" I don't want to give a false impression. It can look so easy, when you have a baby nurse, and a nanny, a helpful husband, and you don't really have to worry about cleaning the house. My best advice is, don't set unrealistic expectations—set a low bar.

SPOTLIGHT ON . . .

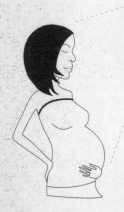

Salli Richardson Whitfield will tell you that when she's pregnant she's showing off her belly 99.9 percent of the time. It's bad enough that she's beautiful, and married to the very yummy D'ondre Whitfield; the least she could do is get one stretch mark to make the rest of us feel good. No chance. She also likes to shoot from the hip, ride motorcycles, and tell it like it is. Nothing like the quiet and love-starved wife she played in Antwone Fisher. *She represents the new breed of over-thirty-five moms—healthy, sexy, and ready for motherhood.*

In retrospect, as a mother I wish I would have done it a little earlier [she had her first baby at age thirty-six] so that I could have more than two kids before I hit a really high-risk age. Now I only have time for one more in two years. But I did it at the perfect time for me. I've done everything I wanted to do. Babies take a lot of patience. And careers take a long time to develop. You may not be ready at thirty. Right now, I don't feel like I'm missing anything. If my husband wants to go to an industry party or event, I'm like Go ahead, honey, I'm cool right here, and I'm really comfortable with that. Now we stay home most of the time. I know lots of our mothers did it by themselves, but, good Lord, it's hard. My husband always says, there's a reason why it takes two to make them, because it takes two to raise them.

My pregnancy went really well. I had the amniocentesis, and I was much more relaxed after that. I didn't get sick and I was really active. I walked about four miles a day, and I did prenatal yoga twice a week. When I got bigger, I started swimming, doing about forty laps a day. In fact, my water broke in yoga class. I had gas, so that was fun. To avoid constipation I drank a glass of prune juice every morning, and one cup of coffee every day to help keep me clean. I figured one cup a day wouldn't hurt.

I didn't have a lot of cravings, but my husband and I had a rule: If I wanted ice cream, I definitely gave in, but I had to work for it. The 31 Flavors is two miles away, and if I wanted it I had to walk there and get it and walk back.

During the pregnancy I used BabyPlus—it's a preeducational

device that allows the baby to hear different variants of the sound of a heartbeat. Each sound is a different lesson, where the baby learns how to differentiate between the different sounds. It is meant to stimulate the development of extra cells in the fetal brain and raise their IQ and make their neck stronger, a lot of stuff. You do it for one hour in the morning and one hour in the evening. And now my baby is very mellow, she holds up her neck like a much older baby, and she's calm. I'd definitely recommend that to other moms-to-be.

One of my biggest pregnancy hurdles was accepting weight gain. I've never been fat in my life. In the beginning, there was a phase where people didn't know I was pregnant and I just looked chubby. After I got over those feelings and actually looked pregnant, I felt sexy all the time. Everything on me was tight. My stomach was always out and my skin looked really good. My father was like "Do you go everywhere with your stomach out?" And I said, "Yes." I loved to wear a little skirt under my tummy and a tube top. And I loved spending money on cute maternity clothes. If you look miserable you feel miserable. And I must say, I was a fabulous pregnant woman.

My labor plan involved hypno-birthing, where I learned how to bring myself into a deep state of meditation. Three or four hours would go by and I never moved. D'ondre learned to say things to keep me in that relaxed state. My mom was there, so every now and then I'd pop an eye open, and say, "Are you okay, Ma?" She said, "I'm okay," and I'd go right back into my trance. I had off-the-charts contractions for five hours straight, with no breaks. I ended up having an epidural, but I would have never made it through fourteen hours of labor without the hypno-birthing techniques.

My best pregnancy advice is definitely exercise. Yoga and walking, both can strengthen you for the pregnancy and help your stamina for labor. Also I started working out again right after the baby because the body has memory, and the longer you wait, the harder it will be. And when people want to tell you their pregnancy horror stories, tell them to shut up. That does not have to be your experience. Only listen to the pleasant experiences.

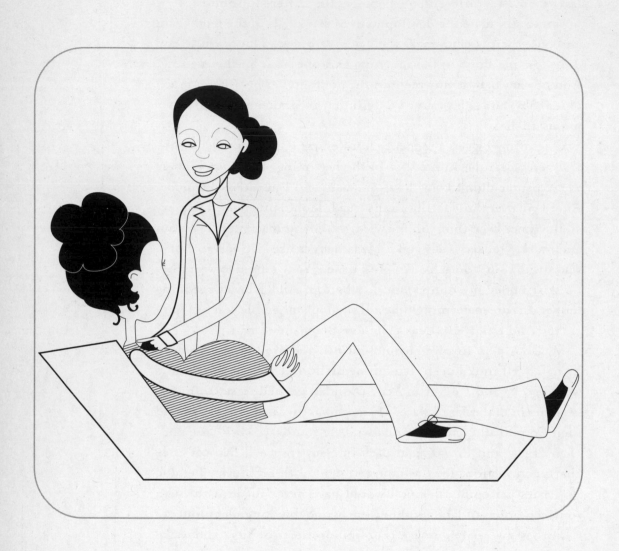

6

Seven Medical Conditions That More Commonly Affect Black Women and What to Do During Pregnancy

Black women are hit with more than their fair share of health problems. At times, our genes, diet, and lifestyle are the culprits. Other times there is no readily visible source. Either way, if you have a chronic health problem, it doesn't mean that you can't have a healthy pregnancy or a healthy baby. You may require special care, however. This chapter gives general advice on some of the more common health problems that disproportionately affect black women, how they may affect your pregnancy, and what to do about them. To help answer these questions, we've interviewed distinguished ob-gyns who weigh in on the correct protocol and what lifestyle changes may be necessary to increase your chances for a healthy baby and a healthy you. (Please note: This is only general information. You and your personal doctor should create a plan that is specifically tailored to your needs.)

Meet the Doctors

Gail N. Jackson, M.D.

Dr. Gail Jackson is a Hollywood staple. With over fifteen years of experience, Dr. Jackson has a very successful private practice in Beverly Hills, located in the Cedars-Sinai Medical Towers. She is an active member of the medical staff of Cedars-Sinai Hospital. A graduate of Howard University College of Medicine, she has served as past president of the Association of Black Women Physicians and has taken her expertise to remote villages in West Africa as a volunteer doctor.

Andrea M. Jackson, M.D.

Dr. Andrea Jackson (no relation to Dr. Gail Jackson, just a popular black folks' name) is a graduate of Tufts University and the Duke University School of Medicine. After eleven years in private practice, Dr. Jackson joined the Physician and Midwife Collaborative Practice in Alexandria, Virginia, which has eight doctors and seven board-certified midwives. The collaborative practice offers the expertise of physicians along with the one-on-one personal attention of midwives. Dr. Jackson is trained in high-risk and low-risk obstetrics, and her work includes integrating alternative and traditional therapies.

Geddis Abel-Bey, M.D.

Dr. Geddis Abel-Bey is a board-certified ob-gyn who has over twenty-five years of experience and a thriving private practice in Flushing, Queens, New York. A graduate of Cornell University and Howard University College of Medicine, Dr. Abel-Bey is a staff physician at Long Island Jewish Hospital, the New York Hospital Medical Center of Queens, and North Shore University Hospital in Manhasset, New York. He sits on several boards and serves as a district chairman for the American College of Obstetrics and Gynecology and is a past president of the Queens (New York) Ob/Gyn Society.

FIBROIDS

Black women have the highest rates of fibroids—noncancerous tumors of the uterus. It is estimated that 50 to 75 percent of black women have fibroids. They can be found on the surface of the uterus, within its walls, or in the uterine cavity. Women can have fibroids in one location or all three. Black women are also more likely to have severe pain, anemia, and larger and more numerous fibroids than women of other racial groups. Although individual family genetics may play a role, studies show that women of African descent who live in other countries do not appear to have as high an incidence of fibroids. To some, this suggests that diet or other environmental factors are at work in the development of fibroids in black women in America. Dr. Andrea Jackson has another theory. "We know that estrogen is produced in fatty tissue; therefore people who have more fat have higher estrogen levels. We also know that estrogen is related to fibroids, so it is logical and plausible that women who are overweight have a higher rate of fibroids and more fibroid growth. Since we also know that fibroids are linked to hormones, it seems logical that avoiding meats and chicken with hormones in it may also be a help."

Managing Your Pregnancy

Women who have fibroids can still have a normal pregnancy and vaginal delivery. "Location, location, location, is key with fibroids. I've seen women with a fibroid the size of a cantaloupe that appears to sit on top of the uterus like a top hat. This fibroid may not complicate the pregnancy and delivery. If the fibroids block the cervix, then that is a different matter, as this may inhibit the ability to deliver vaginally. Women need to know that the presence of fibroids doesn't mean you can't get pregnant or have a healthy pregnancy," says Dr. Gail Jackson.

Fibroid tumors may grow (as a result of the increased levels of estrogen), remain the same, or shrink during pregnancy, but most studies show that in the majority of cases they don't significantly increase in size during pregnancy. However, a small percentage of tumors may more than double in size. Sometimes these fast-growing tumors can outgrow their blood supply and begin to degenerate, a problem called "red degeneration." The degeneration causes severe pain and occasionally light vaginal bleeding, along with vomiting, nausea, and a low-grade fever. The pain, which occurs over the spot where the fibroid is situated, may radiate down the back and usually begins in the second trimester at around twenty weeks. "If the pain is severe, it can stimulate the uterus to start contracting. This can cause preterm labor. In that case you may be hospitalized or put on bed rest until all signs of preterm labor are gone," says Dr. Gail Jackson. The frequent pain also causes confusion in pregnancy—is it the fibroids or preterm labor?—so women who have fibroids find themselves at the doctor's office more frequently, notes Dr. Abel-Bey. But there is no need to worry that your fibroids will hurt or deform a baby. "There's probably one case in an old obstetrics textbook, but it is so rare that it is not worth thinking about," says Dr. Andrea Jackson. However, you may look much larger than another woman at the same point in her pregnancy. "Be prepared for comments about how big you look, etc., and don't let them bother you," Dr. Andrea Jackson says.

Risks: Depending on their locations, fibroids can sometimes increase the risk of miscarriage during the first and second trimesters or increase the chance of preterm labor. The most serious complications occur when the placenta grows near or over the surface of a fibroid inside the uterus. In these cases, the growing baby can be deprived of sufficient nutrients and have a low birth weight, the membrane may rupture prematurely, or in some cases, fibroids can also obstruct the birth canal, complicating labor and delivery.

If fibroids lead to preterm labor, your doctor will likely recommend bed rest. If severe bleeding occurs, the treatment may include hospitalization, monitoring of the baby's condition, and, if needed, a blood transfusion. Surgery for removing fibroids is avoided during pregnancy, because it can lead to preterm delivery and excessive blood loss.

Fibroids do not prevent you from delivering vaginally. However, your risk of having a cesarean delivery may also increase if your fibroids are in the lower part of the uterus, because there they can block the baby's descent, or if you have several fibroids, which can prevent the uterus from contracting properly and progressing in labor.

Postpartum Care: After delivery, the fibroids may trigger significant bleeding, making iron supplements or even a blood transfusion necessary postpartum. If your fibroids grew during pregnancy, they may shrink back to their prepregnancy size within a few months after delivery. Dr. Gail Jackson suggests asking friends and family to donate blood ahead of time and have it on order, just in case a postpartum hemorrhage occurs.

High Blood Pressure

Also known as just "pressure" in the black community, hypertension is more common in our community than in the general population. It can be caused by heredity, diet, obesity, or a diet that includes too much salt or too much alcohol. High blood pressure must be treated. It can lead to heart attack, stroke, kidney failure, and premature death.

Managing Your Pregnancy

With close observation and careful management, most women who have high blood pressure can have healthy pregnancies. "You have to keep your blood pressure under control during pregnancy," says Dr. Gail Jackson. Chronic hypertension can significantly worsen during pregnancy and cause serious problems for you and your baby. In order to monitor the baby's health and development carefully, frequent visits and repeated ultrasounds are typically done to gauge fetal growth and the baby's blood flow distribution. Dr. Andrea Jackson warns that blood pressure typically lowers somewhat on its own during the second trimester. "This is not a sign to lose vigilance, because it typically goes back up in the third trimester," she says.

In most cases, women who have high blood pressure will need to deliver a few weeks before their due date to prevent complications. Before that, you will likely see your doctor more frequently, perhaps every two weeks until the third trimester, when the visits will be weekly. At each visit your blood pressure will be taken, and your urine will be checked for excess protein or sugar. Since urinary tract infections are common in hypertensive women, your urine may also be periodically tested for bacteria. Your own doctor may be assisted by a high-risk pregnancy specialist, called a *perinatologist.*

Dr. Abel-Bey also recommends seeing a nutritionist. "The things that led you to have high blood pressure are probably diet-related. I can tell you to throw the salt shaker out the window and put the smoked meats away, but I can't follow you home. You have to learn to eat better for you, your baby, and hopefully for your lifetime," he says. Other advice for a successful pregnancy includes reducing stress and limiting work hours. Dr. Gail Jackson suggests preparing yourself for the strong possibility of being on bed rest in the third trimester.

The good news is that many blood pressure medications have been used some thirty years and have been proved safe and effective during pregnancy, according to Dr. Gail Jackson.

Risks: The most dangerous pregnancy complication of high blood pressure is preeclampsia, a condition whose symptoms include headaches, swelling, blurred vision, abdominal pain, and sudden weight gain. Your baby faces the risk of growth impairment, a greater risk the placenta will separate from the uterus before labor (placental abruption), and possible side effects from medications used to treat the mother's hypertension, such as a breathing problem. Some studies have shown that these risks are greatest for women over forty who have had hypertension for more than fifteen years. You, the mother, are at risk for congestive heart failure, seizures, kidney or liver malfunctioning, vision changes, and stroke. If the problem becomes severe, it can be life-threatening.

Diabetes

Diabetes is a disease that affects the regulation of blood sugar (glucose), the body's main source of energy. Typically, the foods you eat are broken down to glucose and absorbed into the bloodstream minutes to hours later. Insulin, a hormone secreted by the pancreas, then helps glucose enter your cells for energy use or storage. In people who have diabetes, this process doesn't function properly. If your pancreas doesn't produce enough insulin or if your body is unable to use the insulin that it does produce effectively, diabetes or "sugar" can develop. Instead of going into the cells, the glucose accumulates in the bloodstream and is eventually passed in the urine. According to recent data from the Centers for Disease Control, diabetes affects more than 16 million adults and children in the United States and is twice as common among black women as white women. Their data show that 2.3 million (10.8 percent) of non-Hispanic blacks suffer from diabetes. It tends to run in families and obesity puts you in a higher risk category for development of the disease.

The two major categories of diabetes are type I and type II. People who have type I diabetes have to have insulin injections on a regular basis to control their disease. Those who have type II, the more common variation among black women, don't usually need insulin and can control the disease with a strict diet and exercise and sometimes medications.

Women who have diabetes should plan their pregnancies carefully, with a goal of gaining the best control of the disease before conception. In fact, prepregnancy counseling is highly recommended, according to Dr. Abel-Bey.

Managing Your Pregnancy

Remember: your baby's glucose level is directly tied to yours. When yours is high, so is your baby's. In fact, studies show that the rate of birth defects and complications is directly related to a woman's control of her blood sugar in the early stages after conception and the first trimester, according to Dr. Andrea Jackson. "You need absolutely excellent blood sugar control," she says.

Your doctor may recommend that you increase your insulin dosage because hormones from the placenta can hinder the normal response to insulin. Some women may need two to three times their usual does of insulin to control their blood sugar. Women who have had retinopathy, an eye complication brought on by diabetes, should see an ophthalmologist because pregnancy can cause retinopathy to worsen. The National Institute of Diabetes and Digestive and Kidney Diseases (NIDDK) notes that African Americans are 40 to 50 percent more likely than whites to have diabetic retinopathy. If you have severe nausea and vomiting, you may have difficulty maintaining a proper diet—one of the keys to a successful pregnancy with diabetes—and you may experience hypoglycemia, or low blood sugar. Hypoglycemia may be caused by delaying or skipping a meal, taking too much insulin, or eating too little food. Your doctor will also likely review your medications, since some oral medications may pose a risk of birth defects.

Since women who have diabetes have a greater risk of having a baby who has neural tube defects, your baby's development will be frequently monitored. An alpha-fetoprotein (AFP) blood test is recommended to check for defects in the neural tube. Dr. Abel-Bey recommends more frequent sonograms to track the baby's growth, to measure the amount of amniotic fluid, and to check for heart defects.

Beyond the doctor visits and frequent tests, it all comes down to you. You are the only one who can ensure the healthiest baby possible. "A diabetic woman must closely adhere to the recommended diet. These forty weeks require a significant commitment to your health and the health of your baby. Respect that commitment," says Dr. Gail Jackson. Monitoring your sugar levels, keeping accurate records, as well as maintaining a diary of the foods you eat and the amount of medication you take are critical.

Risks: If you have diabetes and your blood sugar levels are kept under control before conception and during pregnancy, you have a strong chance of having a healthy pregnancy and delivering a healthy baby. If the diabetes is not under control, you can have a higher risk of having a baby who has a birth defect of the brain or spinal cord, kidneys, or heart. You are also at a higher risk for miscarriage and stillbirth. Even when the disease is well managed, there is an increased risk of preterm labor, kidney and urinary tract infections, preeclampsia (pregnancy-related high blood pressure), excess amniotic fluid, and hypertension. If the diabetes is not under control in the early stages of pregnancy when the organs are forming, your baby can have defects of the heart, skeleton, kidneys, central nervous system, and digestive system.

You are also at risk for having a baby who weighs ten pounds or more if your diabetes is not under control. That's because when the levels of blood sugar become too high, the baby receives a very high glucose intake and produces extra insulin to break down the sugar and store the fat. The fat tends to accumulate and cause a baby to be larger than normal. This medical condition is called macrosomia. Your doctor will likely monitor your baby's growth closely to check for any warning signs of this condition or other effects of the diabetes. Large babies are more likely to be delivered by C-section to avoid a condition called shoulder distotia, in which labor doesn't progress, and the baby cannot be delivered, because his or her shoulder is stuck in the birth canal. Other less severe birth injuries such as a broken collarbone or nerve damage to the arm can occur.

Labor is often induced before the baby reaches full term in pregnancies when the diabetes is not under control, because of the risk of stillbirth. An early birth can create another problem. Babies born to women who have diabetes are prone to development of respiratory distress syndrome and jaundice.

Overweight/Obesity

According to the American Cancer Society, the nation's proportion of overweight adults is 61 percent, but among black women the rate is much higher—77 percent. Obesity is determined by measurement of body fat, not merely body weight. People might be over the weight limit for normal standards, but if they are very muscular and have low body fat, they are not obese. Others might be normal or underweight but still have excessive body fat. The most commonly used gauge of obesity is the body mass index (BMI). You can figure out your BMI with the following steps.

1. Multiply your weight in pounds by 703.
2. Divide that answer by your height in inches.
3. Divide that number again by your height in inches.

For example, a woman who weighs 150 pounds and is five feet eight inches (or 68 inches) tall has a BMI of 22.8. In general, the federal guidelines say, a BMI of 25 to 29.9 means you're overweight and a BMI of 30 and above is defined as obese. Some evidence suggests that whites have the lowest obesity rate, at a BMI of 24.3 to 24.7; and African Americans are better off in the range of 26.8 to 27.1. However, studies also show that 50 percent of blacks are overweight. In pregnancy, being overweight or obese can lead to pregnancy complications and a difficult labor and delivery. The risk for a pregnant woman of being hospitalized goes up four times if she's overweight. If her BMI is over 35, the risk increases six or seven times, according to Dr. Abel-Bey. Obesity also raises your likeihood of development of diabetes, hypertension, heart disease, and some cancers.

Managing Your Pregnancy

Ideally, every overweight woman should have preconception counseling and a physical prior to conception. If possible, doctors will recommend reaching a more average weight several months before conceiving, as this will help reduce your risks of complications. However, do not diet if you are already pregnant; you should be on the same two-thousand-calorie-per-day diet as any other woman, says Dr. Gail Jackson. "This [dieting] is not at all recommended during pregnancy and you will not look significantly larger because you are pregnant. And there are plenty of flattering maternity clothes for plus size women," she says.

You will likely be referred to a nutritionist who can help you get all of the necessary nutrients and adopt a healthier eating lifestyle. "This is a major issue in black America. There is not enough knowledge about what is a good diet. I would definitely recommend a nutritionist to help her make better eating choices," says Dr. Andrea Jackson. "An overweight woman has to focus on what they call a nutrient-dense diet. Foods that are nutrient dense, such as whole grains, beans, vegetables, low-fat dairy, and lean protein, provide a high nutrient-to-calorie ratio. Foods with low nutrient density have a lot of fat and sugar but basically no other nutrients," says Dr. Abel-Bey.

Your physician will also closely monitor your weight gain and general health during pregnancy and may ask you to limit your weight gain to fifteen to twenty pounds, which basically equals the weight of the baby, placenta, added blood volume and other fluids, and increased breast size. Some women may be advised otherwise, so consult your doctor. For example, Dr. Gail Jackson recommends overweight women put on twenty to twenty-five pounds and encourages small but steady weight gain.

Another problem for overweight women is with sonography. "It is always more difficult because you cannot see the baby as clearly so you are more likely to miss something. All of the typical in-office measurements and the hands-on methods of checking the size of uterus and how well the baby is growing are less accurate. You can't really trust it," says Dr. Andrea Jackson.

Risks: Overweight women have an increased risk of having babies who have birth defects, particularly neural tube defects, such as spina bifida. There is also a greater risk of delivering their babies late and of development of hypertension, diabetes, and gallbladder disease. The March of Dimes Task Force on Nutrition and Optimal Human Development presented a report showing that women who are overweight or obese are 30 to 40 percent more likely to have a baby who has major birth defects such as those that affect the brain, heart, and digestive system. Folic acid supplements, which are usually effective in preventing these conditions, may not be as protective in overweight women, according to some studies. Preeclampsia (high blood pressure, swelling, and protein in your urine) is seen more frequently in obese women and can lead to seizures, premature delivery, fetal distress, and death. The higher rate of complications also makes you more likely to have labor induced or to have a C-section. When an overweight woman has a C-section, complications related to anesthesia, wound infections, and life-threatening pulmonary embolus (a blockage of an artery in the lungs by fat, air, tumor tissue, or blood clot) are generally more common.

Babies of obese women run a higher risk of being large—nine pounds or more—and can sustain injuries during vaginal delivery. Your baby also runs a greater risk of neural tube defects, according to Dr. Gail Jackson. Obese women often have medical conditions such as high blood pressure that can cause intrauterine growth retardation and low birth weight. The effect of your weight on your child doesn't end at birth. In a study of African American children, having an overweight pregnant mother increased a child's risk for being overweight later in life.

LUPUS

Lupus is a chronic inflammatory disease of several organ systems and can affect the skin, kidneys, joints, blood cells, heart, and lungs. The body's immune system normally makes proteins called antibodies to protect the body against viruses, bacteria, and other foreign materials. These foreign materials are called antigens. With lupus, the immune system loses its ability to tell the difference between foreign substances (antigens) and its own cells and tissues. The immune system then makes antibodies directed against itself—the body basically attacks its own organs. These antibodies, called *autoantibodies,* react with the "self" antigens to form immune complexes. The immune complexes build up in the tissues and can cause inflammation, injury to tissues, and pain. There is no cure for lupus, and people who have it experience painful "flares" of the symptoms.

The disease affects about 14 million Americans; about 90 percent of those are women. Black women are three times more likely to have lupus than white women, according to the U.S. Department of Health. And we have much higher mortality rates related to the disease.

However, successful pregnancies are possible. Research shows that more than 50 percent of all pregnancies of women who have lupus are successful, 25 percent deliver normal babies prematurely, and miscarriage or fetal death accounts for less than 20 percent of all pregnancies, according to the Lupus Foundation of America.

Most babies born to a mother who has lupus do not have the disease. However, about 33 percent of people who have lupus have an antibody known as the anti-Ro, or anti-SSA, antibody. About 10 percent of women who have anti-Ro antibodies and about 3 percent of all women who have lupus will have a baby who has a syndrome called neonatal lupus. This is the only congenital abnormality found in children of mothers who have lupus, and it consists of a rash that goes away, a low blood platelet count that returns to normal over time, and a heartbeat abnormality. Though rare and permanent, the heartbeat abnormality is treatable, usually with a pacemaker to regulate the baby's heartbeat. Babies who have this abnormality do tend to grow normally.

Managing Your Pregnancy

Some women who have lupus actually experience an improvement in their disease symptoms when pregnant. If the lupus is active during pregnancy, about half of women experience a worsening of their condition. However, women who are symptom free at the time of conception have a good chance for a healthy baby and pregnancy. Women who conceive after five to six months of remission are less likely to experience a flare-up during pregnancy. "The response in pregnancy varies wildly from no effect at all to a high risk of recurrent miscarriage, poor fetal growth, placental abruption, and stillbirth. Also, be prepared for a lupus flare-up to six weeks after a delivery or miscarriage. Still, I've seen good, successful pregnancies with women with lupus," says Dr. Andrea Jackson.

All lupus pregnancies are considered "high risk," so unless your ob-gyn has particular expertise in this area, she will likely comanage your care with a high-risk pregnancy specialist or perinatologist. You will have more scheduled office visits and more testing to monitor your baby's growth and your lupus. By closely monitoring you, your doctor can distinguish the symptoms of a lupus flare-up from the normal body changes that occur during pregnancy. For example, because the ligaments that hold the joints together normally soften in pregnancy, fluid may accumulate in the joints (especially in the knees) and cause swelling. Although this condition suggests inflammation due to lupus, it may simply be the swelling that occurs during a normal pregnancy.

Dr. Andrea Jackson recommends extra sonograms to monitor

the growth of the baby and to make sure there is adequate blood flow through the cord, particularly in the third trimester. She also advises a nonstress test to check for healthy heart patterns and a biophysical profile (which includes an ultrasound and nonstress test) of the baby in the latter part of the third trimester.

Many women can deliver vaginally, if they have been carefully monitored and the lupus is without symptoms. However, doctors will likely advise you not to be overly committed to the idea of a "natural" delivery.

Risks: If you have active lupus during your pregnancy, you are at a higher risk of miscarriage, stillbirth, or other pregnancy complications. You are also at risk of development of high blood pressure or preeclampsia, especially if your kidneys have been affected by the disease. Your baby may have poor fetal growth or an unusually low heart rate, which is also known as fetal heart block. During the second trimester, you will likely have a test called a fetal cardiac echo, which shows how your baby's heart is developing and performing.

About one in three, or 33 percent of women who have lupus, have antibodies that can interfere with the functioning of the placenta. These antibodies can cause blood clots in the placenta that prevent it from growing and functioning normally. The blood clots tend to occur during the second trimester. Since the placenta is the means by which the baby is fed and receives vital nourishment, this condition can slow the baby's growth. Your doctor can advise you of the various treatments available, including early delivery or medication.

Human Immunodeficiency Virus

Studies show that the human immunodeficiency virus (HIV) rate of childbearing black women is twenty-three times that of white women. According to the Centers for Disease Control, in 2000, HIV/acquired immunodeficiency syndrome (AIDS) was among the top three causes of death for African American women aged thirty-five to forty-four. Although blacks represent roughly 13 percent of the nation's population, CDC's data show that we account for 39 percent—or about 347,000—of the 886,000 AIDS cases diagnosed since the beginning of the epidemic. By December 2002 more than 185,000 blacks had died of AIDS. Sixty-two percent of all children born to HIV/AIDS-infected mothers were African American. There is no doubt that HIV/AIDS is devastating the black community. But many women are not diagnosed because they don't fit their own idea of who is at high risk of the disease.

Managing Your Pregnancy

Pregnancy has no effect on the progress of the HIV infection. It neither increases nor decreases the chance that HIV will develop into AIDS. You will likely be referred to an infectious disease specialist who has expertise in HIV pregnancies, and will also be seen by a high-risk pregnancy specialist (perinatologist), and possibly a dentist and ophthalmologist. You will be advised as to the best course of medicines that can slow the progress of the disease and fight off infection. Dr. Abel-Bey says that an infectious disease specialist is key since your compromised immune system and pregnancy make you more susceptible to disease. "The specialist will also make sure you don't have any other illnesses," he says.

The generally accepted protocol for minimizing the risk of transmission to your baby involves taking antiretroviral medications like ZDV (or zidovudine, also known as AZT) after the first three to four months of pregnancy. In most cases, at or after the fourteenth week of pregnancy, women are given ZDV, which they continue and are given during labor—this is in line with the recent recommendations by the U.S. Public Health Service. ZDV is not taken at the start of pregnancy, because its safety when taken so early in gestation is not clear. In 1994, AZT became the first drug used to prevent HIV transmission, and it remains the only drug thoroughly studied for use during pregnancy.

Studies also show that some HIV-infected women can reduce the risk of transmission by 50 percent by having a C-section delivery before labor begins and their membranes rupture. A 1999 study by the National Institute of Child Health and Human Development found that only 2 percent of women who took HIV-fighting drugs in pregnancy and had a C-section passed the virus on to their baby, compared to 7.3 percent who took the medications but did not have a C-section. The American College of Obstetricians and Gynecologists recommends a C-section at thirty-eight weeks, unless the mother has undetectable amounts of virus in the blood.

"Do things that boost the immune system—have a healthy diet; get plenty of rest; if feasible, exercise to strengthen your body; and reduce the stress in your life. Stress can take a big toll on the immune system," advises Dr. Andrea Jackson.

Risks: The major risk is that of passing an infection to your baby during pregnancy, labor (via your blood and vaginal secretions), or breast-feeding. About 15 percent of HIV-infected babies exhibit serious signs and symptoms of the disease or die in the first year of life. Close to half don't live past age ten. Although there is no cure for HIV, there are treatments now available that can significantly reduce a mother's risk of passing HIV to her baby. Your medical treatment is critical in influencing the risk of transmission. A government study in 1994 showed that drug treatment during pregnancy greatly reduces the risk that an HIV-infected mother will pass the virus to her baby. Between 1992 and 1999, the number of children reported to the CDC who had contracted HIV from their mother declined by 83 percent. These days, new treatments are such that the rate of transmission has been reduced to 2 percent or less, according to the March of Dimes.

Your doctor can also make sure your baby is promptly tested for infection after birth. When infants test positive early, they can be given HIV-fighting drugs that have been proven to slow the progression of the disease and improve survival rates.

SICKLE CELL

Sickle-cell disease is a blood disorder, passed down from parents to children. It is the most common genetic disorder of African Americans. "All African American women should be screened for sickle cell. Physicians notoriously fail to do this and it is one of my pet peeves. It is essential because sickle cell is very prevalent in all people of color, from American blacks, to Caribbeans, to people of Mediterranean descent. Be very proactive in obtaining your sickle cell status. Be tested for all the variants of the disease," advises Dr. Andrea Jackson.

Normal red blood cells are round and smooth and can move through the blood vessels easily. Sickle cells are hard and elongated and have a curved edge and a crescentlike shape. These cells cannot squeeze through small blood vessels. When the oxygen level is low, such as when the body is fighting infection, the cells become stiff and stick together, clogging the blood vessels. They block the organs from getting needed blood. Blocked blood vessels and damaged organs can cause acute, painful episodes. These painful "crises," which occur in almost all sickle cell patients at some point in their life, can last hours to days, affecting the bones of the back and the chest. Some patients have one episode every few years; others have many episodes per year. The crises can be severe enough to require admission to a hospital for pain control and intravenous fluids.

Your body destroys sickle cells quickly, but it can't make new red ones fast enough—this is called anemia. Sickle cell anemia is the most serious type of sickle cell disease. It can cause pain and swelling of the hands and feet, fatigue, shortness of breath, yellow color in the skin and eyes, and pain in any organ or joint. Every year, about one in four hundred African Americans is born with sickle cell anemia.

Another form of sickle cell disease is sickle C disease. This disease occurs when you inherit a protein that helps transport oxygen from the lungs to all parts of the body, hemoglobin S, from one parent and hemoglobin C from the other parent (hemoglobin C is an abnormal hemoglobin found in about two of every one hundred blacks). The presence of sickle C disease can result in life-threatening lung complications at or around the time of delivery, according to Dr. Gail Jackson.

Even if you don't have sickle cell disease, you may carry the trait. Some studies estimate that one in twelve blacks has the sickle cell trait. That is why being tested for the type of hemoglobin you have and being screened for the sickle cell disease or the trait is so important. If your blood shows an abnormality, then the father will have to be tested as well. If you, but not the father, have the trait, you can generally have a normal pregnancy with no health problems. If you both have the trait, there is a one-in-four chance your child will be born with the disease. "People with sickle cell are now living to the age where they can bear children. Their children could very well do the same or better," says Dr. Andrea Jackson.

Managing Your Pregnancy

There is a lot you and your doctor can do to make sure you have a healthy baby. "It can be managed successfully but it does require a high level of expertise," says Dr. Andrea Jackson. First, you will need a high-risk pregnancy obstetrician (perinatologist) and a hematologist. "The consultation with the hematologist is important. We know she has one blood problem, and maybe there is another one," says Dr. Abel-Bey.

You will have more frequent prenatal visits, and more frequent blood and urine tests. Dr. Gail Jackson says it is important to check for any bacteria in the urine. "We treat any sign of infection quickly to prevent it from reaching up to the bladder and kidneys, which can cause preterm labor," she says. Even at your first prenatal visit, your initial tests may include a complete blood count, hemoglobin electrophoresis (for your partner as well), liver function tests, a test for hepatitis B and C, blood group and antibody typing, a test for rubella antibodies, and a syphilis test.

Pregnant women who have sickle cell are almost always anemic at the first prenatal visit. Sickle cell patients may be overloaded with iron because of frequent past transfusions, so you may be advised to avoid iron supplements. Morning sickness poses extra risks for women who have sickle cell, as it can lead to dehydration, and dehydration causes sickle cell crises. Tests for urinary tract infection will be done at each prenatal visit, as women who have sickle cell are at increased risk for infection. During the last trimester you may have additional fetal testing. Anemia is likely to be most severe during the final months of pregnancy and may require blood transfusions. In labor and delivery, your team of specialists will take special care to prevent a crisis. Vaginal delivery is preferred since there is a higher risk of blood loss, infection, and blood clots with a C-section. After delivery, you will likely be advised to drink a lot of fluids to prevent dehydration. Also you should take special care of any stitches or incision areas to prevent infection.

Risks: Women who are pregnant and have sickle cell have more frequent sickle cell crises because of the extra stress of pregnancy. Pregnancy is an intense burden on a woman's body, and this incredible strain can easily exacerbate the sickling of red blood cells. A sickle crisis will occur in about a third of pregnancies. When these cells cluster together, they can build up in various organs throughout the body, leading to intense pain. Furthermore, because blood vessels can become blocked, body tissues may be deprived of their oxygen and die. When this happens, the body's first response is to send blood to the most important organs in the body—and the uterus isn't one of them—in order to survive, so if a woman is pregnant, her sickle cell anemia can deprive her fetus of oxygen and nutrients.

Even with the best medical care, some significant risks remain. During pregnancy, infections can occur more frequently and lead to painful crises. These infections may include urinary tract infection, pneumonia, and uterine infection. Pregnant women who have sickle cell are at higher risk of miscarriage, premature labor, preeclampsia, and cesarean section. In addition, the fetuses are more likely to have growth lags and more trouble with the stresses of labor and delivery. The risk of stillbirth or low birth-weight is also increased. After the birth, all women are more likely to have infections and blood clots, but the risk for sickle cell mothers is even greater.

Spotlight On . . .

Ever since Essence *magazine hit the scene in 1970, black women have had a magazine to call their own. Competitors come and go, but* Essence *remains the country's most successful black women's magazine. Michelle Ebanks can take a little credit for that; as president of Essence Communications Partners, she oversees circulation, production, advertising, marketing, and new ventures. That doesn't leave much time for eating lunch, let alone having a baby. But somehow Michelle managed two—born seventeen months apart. She had her first at age thirty-nine. Sitting in her spacious New York City office, overlooking the buzz, lights, and lure of Times Square, Michelle shares her thoughts on job anxiety, being pregnant on 9/11, and why she'll never trust a doctor quite as much again.*

I'm going to tell my story backward because the most important thing a pregnant woman should know is that you must be your own health advocate. I learned this through an eye-opening experience. I was ten days past my due date with my first child and my doctor continued to tell me not to worry. But I went on the Internet and saw some research that said there is a higher risk of a stillbirth when you are overdue. That freaked me out. At my next appointment the doctor did a stress test, said we were both fine, and was about to send me home. But I happened to ask the technician what other tests were important at this stage, and she mentioned one that measured your amniotic fluid level. My husband and I asked if we could have that test. It showed my fluid was dangerously low, which is what can cause stillbirths. They wouldn't let me go home. I went to Labor & Delivery immediately.

Later at the hospital, my husband and I asked the nurse why the line disappeared on the baby's heartbeat monitor whenever I had a contraction. She panicked, ran for the doctor, who yelled at her for not noticing it sooner. The baby was in distress because of the low fluid. In ten seconds, the delivery room turned into an operating room. It was traumatic. I learned to never turn over ultimate responsibility of your and your baby's life to the doctor. What if we never asked those questions? No matter how many degrees they have, or how much you would like to trust them, you really cannot.

It seems that much of my pregnancy experience has been eventful. I was five months pregnant on 9/11. We were in a meeting and the CFO came down the hall and told us a plane hit the World Trade Center. We gathered around the TV. And then the second plane hit. There was chaos in the office because people had families there. The trains were down. We were trying to get people home. I'm trying to get in contact with my husband. The streets were chaotic. There was a bomb scare in our building, and I thought, I'm bringing a life into a world that has just turned upside down. That was really scary. You feel through your children. You feel for your children. It hurts to think about how much things have changed in our own lifetime. What is it going to be like for them?

This was a really sobering time when I had been so elated about conceiving after trying for two years. I was so happy and everyone was so happy for me. I had been married to my career; a lot of people didn't think it would ever happen for me.

When it did happen, I had only been at *Essence* for two months. Getting pregnant so soon after starting a new job gave me a lot of anxiety, but after two years of trying, I wasn't going to stop. My pregnancies don't start off well. I had morning sickness all day and then I was completely exhausted. It was a struggle to stay focused and I couldn't tell anyone what was going on. I typically could not make it through the workday. I live fifteen minutes from the office, so I would go home at lunch, sleep for half an hour, and come back. I fell behind with my work. I didn't do as much as I set out to do because I just couldn't. The good news was that I was so new here, people didn't know what to expect of me. But I knew I could do more.

There was also the stress of managing the doctor's appointments, and worrying would I miscarry, while trying to keep eleven- to twelve-hour workdays. I've always been a workaholic. And I didn't know what else to do. I'm the type of person—and I think it is true of most black women—you just deal with it and you get through it.

Exercise used to be my stress outlet. I'd go to the gym four, five times a week before I got pregnant. Then I stopped to be safe during my first trimester. I bought a book on breathing and mediation and used the exercises to alleviate the stress.

The second trimester changed everything for me. I felt great. I didn't have to rush home for a nap. I was back in action—back in the gym doing some low-impact exercises. My husband and I played tennis competitively every weekend like we did before. I felt better than at any other point in my life.

We decided against the amniocentesis, but we did have an alternative test that involves blood work, ultrasounds, and an examination. Two of the blood tests came back positive, and one came back negative, which was very stressful. Since then, I've learned that this is not so unusual because there's wide range of error with this test. But at the time it was difficult. They basically said there could be a chance of a chromosomal abnormality and they offered us the amnio. But again, it took me two years to get pregnant, so I didn't want a 2 percent risk of a miscarriage, so my husband and I talked about it. I remember looking at the doctors, looking at my husband, thinking about my age, and being in that higher-risk group for Down's syndrome. Finally, my husband said, "Let's not have the amnio. We'll be fine." He said, "Besides, you're not that bright anyway, so if our child has a problem . . ." It was great because he completely defused the situation with his British wit. He's been wonderful even through the process of trying to get pregnant. "I didn't marry our children. I married you," he said. I did not have the amnio and we didn't think about it again. Of course, at each ultrasound examination, we paid close attention to the head size and those tests kept on coming back normal, normal, normal. The issue just sort of went away.

The second pregnancy was better in that I don't really remember it because I was so busy with the first child. He always wanted to be held. It was a real challenge. My healthy eating habits slipped and I got dehydrated. My sinuses and eyes dried out and there was a burning pain. Meanwhile, I was busier than ever at work, but during the first trimester, of course, I didn't want to tell anyone. It took me a long time to get pregnant and I don't believe in traveling in my first trimester. But there were a number of trips I needed to take. You can't say "No" without an explanation. It was very stressful.

My best advice: Always take care of yourself. You take care of anyone else, if you're not well. When I practice that to the letter, it makes all the difference in the world.

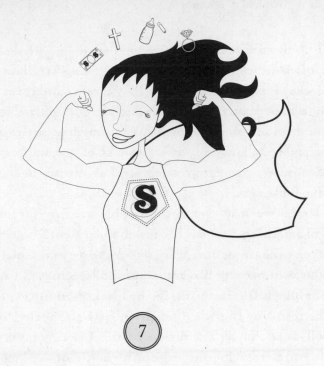

7

Managing Stress and the Strong Black Woman Syndrome in Pregnancy

There are a few things in life that are certain for a black woman in America: stress and more stress. That's because in our society we are hit with the double whammy—black and female. We face both racist and sexist misconceptions in this world. Still, we have accomplished so much. We are leading top organizations, have broken barriers in sports, politics, law, finance, and the arts. College-educated black women already earn more than the median for all working black men, and the rising pay of black women has been credited as the key driver in the creation of America's new black middle class. We have raised the bar of what is acceptable to us in life, career, and love. Yet, for all of our achievements and hard work, we still get no love. We are often misunderstood by mainstream media—portrayed as sassy maids, smart-talking fishwives, abusers of the welfare system, or crackheads. We are rarely celebrated as nurturing mothers and would-be mothers.

At times, we may even feel invisible among our own people. Here's something our parents and the black empowerment rhetoric never prepare us for: class sets us apart and isolates us from even our own people. Black women who've achieved financial success often feel like the misfits of the black community; their career and the resulting lifestyle often are negatively labeled as "bourgie" or "sell-out." There's a divide in the black community. Many women, after carrying the flag in the battle of "us" against them, also wage a "me" against "them" war. A working girl's struggles in corporate America, the misconceptions of the media, and the frustrations of being mistaken for domestic help or a criminal because she lives in a predominantly white neighborhood make her feel pretty low on Official Agenda of Black People.

"If I got shot by a white police officer, I could call Al Sharpton or maybe get some folks together for a protest. But when I'm getting passed over for job promotions and new accounts in favor of underqualified white boys, nobody is making signs or rhyming marching songs for me," says Yvette, a marketing executive from New York.

The complexity of our lives is difficult to bear. Have you ever felt you have to check your real self at the door when you're at work in order to be nonthreatening to white colleagues? Have you ever played down your abilities so as not to outshine black men or to fit in with other black people? There's a word for that—*shifting*—a phrase coined by writer Charisse Jones and Dr. Kumea Shorter-Gooden, based on their research in the African American Women's Voices Project, one of the most comprehensive studies ever conducted of black women's experiences with bias. But before anyone ever put a name on it, we were doing it, as an instinctive survival trait we picked up along the way. Black women are the masters of the shift, stepping in and out of the white world and back into our black community. It's a survival skill most black women have mastered to the point where it is taken for granted. But "shifting" means we don't have the privilege of living our full lives as our true selves. This leads to conflicted feelings along with other psychological problems such as low self-esteem, anxiety, eating disorders, and depression. Basically, it destroys us, body and soul. If it's not the biggies, then there's what psychologists are now calling *micro-insults,* you know, being followed around in the store or being mistaken for the help in a predominantly white neighborhood even if you're wearing a fur coat. No wonder a recent Gallup poll showed that 61 percent of black women said they were dissatisfied with "how blacks are treated in society." The dissatisfaction rate for black men was lower: 47 percent. The same poll also showed that 48 percent of black women, compared to 26 percent of white women, said they were dissatisfied with "how women are treated in society."

Then there are the everyday stresses of life—family, work, children, spouses and significant others, to say nothing of commuter traffic, the creeping line at your favorite java joint, and the unexplainable sky-high price of skinless chicken breasts. It's enough to make you want to scream. But instead, most black women pull out their Strong Black Woman (SBW) persona and suit up. Researchers have studied the different ways men, white women, and black women respond to stress. Men are more likely to take on whatever is causing the stress, or physically or mentally remove themselves from the situation. White women are more likely to have what researchers call a "tend and befriend" response, that is, to devote more time to their kids or seek out support from friends and loved ones. But black women have been noted to tend, befriend, mend, and keep it in.

It's the keeping it in that's the humdinger. After all, studies also prove that black women have more physical responses to stress than white women have. We experience more anxiety, guilt, fear, and restlessness, and less alertness, relaxation, and happiness when faced with psychological stressors. That makes doing the SBW thing downright physically dangerous. Doctors say the frequent or chronic stresses make the body hypervigilant or in a constant state of overdrive, which is damaging to the cardiovascular and gastrointestinal systems.

The legacy of black women in this world is so rooted in hardship that it has become a defining element of the black female experience. Our foremothers are repeatedly portrayed as strong and emotionless creatures who took care of white women, their white children, as well as their own family. When enslaved children and adults were split up and moved to other plantations, it was the slave women who took care of the extended families who remained. In fact, as long as history has documented our existence, we have been taking care of other people. Sometimes we had no other choice, as refusing to do so could mean severe punishment or death. Nor did our foremothers have the luxury of a time-out, bubble bath, or aromatherapy, to help refuel their energy, their spirit, and their soul.

Black women rarely have the luxury of being female, you know, the fairer sex, as society likes to view women. The Bible refers to women as the "weaker vessel," but black women are often denied the perk of being allowed to be weak. In fact, to many of us, a weak black woman is an oxymoron—she simply does not exist. Now, we all have a girlfriend or relative we've labeled as weak for remaining in some unhealthy situation, but chances are that woman has endured something in her life that has eaten away at her self-esteem. Either way, our will to survive is strong.

Back in slavery days, black women were expected to work just as hard as men. For many sisters, that hasn't changed one bit. How many of us would love, even if just for a day, to be a damsel in distress with some knight in shining armor riding in to save us, for a change? Instead, we are often our own knights, forced to save ourselves, our family, and sometimes even our partner. My girlfriend

Sophia and I once had a discussion about our frustration with being cheerleaders—you know, always cheering on everyone else: our siblings, our man, the younger up-and-coming sisters at the job, and the list goes on. But who was there to cheer us on? "Who has the pom-poms out for me?" Sophie asked. "Can a sister get a little rah-rah sometimes?" Many times we can't.

One study looked at women who identified themselves as Strong Black Women and said that identification was an important part of who they were. These women were asked to write a diary detailing their activities and emotions; their blood pressure and heart rate were monitored at the same time. In the diaries, the women did not admit to feeling stressed or were unaware that they were stressed although their blood pressure and heart rate told a different story. Even those who admitted to feeling stressed denied that stress was a problem for them.

Clearly, first we have to work on identifying stress. Then we have to recognize that in the strongest of women, prolonged stress can lead to chronic upper respiratory infections, hypertension, heart disease, and obesity. During pregnancy, stress has been clinically proved to affect birth outcomes adversely. Many experts now conclude that stress causes the release of hormones that weaken the uterus, leading to premature delivery or infant mortality. The hormone changes can occur over a lifetime, not just in pregnancy. They can build up from fear of violence, worries about paying bills, job insecurity, or standing for long periods at work. One study found that pregnancy complications were more frequent among black women who said they were dealing with racial discrimination at work or in housing situations.

For years, health professionals believed that poverty, inadequate prenatal care, and other socioeconomic issues were the root cause of the large gap between the birth outcomes of black women and those of white women. The theory of inadequate prenatal care began to lose water when nearly every state began to offer Medicaid to low-income pregnant women, but there has not yet been a consequential decline in the incidence of low birth weight or infant mortality for blacks. Black women are 2.2 times more likely to have a low-birth-weight infant than their white counterparts. And whereas black infants constitute 17 percent of all births in the United States, they account for 33 percent of all low-birth-weight infants and 38 percent of all very-low-birth-weight infants. Worse yet, the risk of dying of pregnancy-related complications is four times higher for black women than for white women. Until recently, researchers assumed that education, employment, and income provided a shield against poor health and poor birth outcomes for black women. But now it seems that not even education can explain the racial gap in pregnancy outcomes. In fact, the infant mortality rate experienced by black women who are college graduates is *higher* than that of white women who are high school dropouts. And we can't chalk it up to some genetically linked black thing. Babies of black women born in the United States die at a higher rate than those of black immigrant women in similar economic circumstances.

So let's be clear about the message here: Just being a black woman places you in a higher risk category, regardless of whether you are a high school dropout, high school graduate, Harvard M.B.A., or Stanford Ph.D. We are winning the battle to scale corporate ladders, crash through glass ceilings, and gain economic prowess, but we are still losing the war for healthy pregnancies, stronger babies, and fewer complications. And all of the signs point to stress as the main cause.

My big problem with stress is that it has been overcommercialized and simplified into something you can bubble bath away. Or you can just sniff some lavender and you'll be fine. The stress we're talking about is not that kind of stress. There is nothing I can sniff to ease my anxiety about raising a black male in a society that denigrates them. I could soak in a tub until my entire body shriveled up like a prune and still not know how to cope on the job when I work my butt off only to have a young white boy with all the right Daddy credentials slide through and get plum assignments handed to him on a platter. So what we're talking about are the nuances of

racism and sexism that black women take on every day. We're talking about our roles in our families, communities, or church
groups that sap our energy. Before we get started, let's pause for a
reality check.

For as difficult as our lives can be, we have a lot to be grateful
for. Our enslaved ancestors had it much worse. They didn't have
any benefits or maternity leave. In fact, according to historians,
most slaveholders stupidly thought that hard work was healthy and
that a healthy woman would bear more children if she worked
hard, even when pregnant. They clearly didn't have the modern
medical knowledge that shows that overworked pregnant women
not only have a decreased reproductive capacity but also higher
rates of sudden infant death syndrome. Most slave owners viewed
pregnancy as a dilemma that needed to be addressed—how would
they make use of the physical strength of black women while protecting their future investment in them as childbearers? "These
two objectives—one focused on immediate profit returns and the
other on long-term economic considerations—at times clashed, as
women who spent long hours picking cotton, toiling in the fields
with heavy iron hoes, and walking several miles a day sustained
damage to their reproductive systems immediately before and after
giving birth," writes Jacqueline Jones, in *Labor of Love, Labor of Sorrow:
Black Women, Work, and the Family from Slavery to the Present*. "During the
cotton boom years of 1830 to 1860, slave fertility decreased and
miscarriage rates increased due to the heightened demand made
upon women, both in terms of increased workloads in the fields
and family breakups associated with the massed, forced migration
of slaves from the Upper to Lower South," Jones writes.

There were no breaks or special considerations for pregnant
slaves, and some masters had women deliver their children
between the cotton rows. They got their fair share of whipping,
pregnant or not. One historian's account says that pregnant and
nursing mothers were whipped "so that blood and milk flew min-
gled from their breasts." Another report, in *Labor of Love, Labor of
Sorrow*, reveals a method of whipping pregnant women that was used

throughout the South: "They were made to lie face down in a specially dug depression in the ground"—in the sick minds of the slave masters, they were simultaneously protecting the fetus and abusing its mother, as if the two weren't inextricably linked.

The fact that the black race still exists today despite the treatment of its childbearers is in and of itself a testimony to the strength we inherently hold. But feigning strength when you actually feel weakness is dangerous. And stressful.

We are going to examine five key areas of stress. After poring through reams of medical research and speaking to hundreds of black women, I've identified the following key areas or ways of thinking that cause stress. We will examine what's behind them and what you can do about them.

STRONG BLACK WOMAN

There's a nasty myth permeating our community and society that black women are indefatigable, unshakable, and tireless. It's a dangerous myth that has taken root and embedded itself in the psyche of the black community. We are not allowed to be vulnerable. We are not allowed to be needy. That myth is an illusion, a façade that masks a lot of pain and sorrow. We have internalized this myth and made it a truth, but it is not a truth. It is a lie that is destroying black women. It has become a prison that prevents us from living freely; instead we judge ourselves too harshly and we have unrealistic standards. At what cost are we living this lie today? Today our rates of hypertension, depression, and AIDS are skyrocketing. Sisters are breaking under the pressure. Sometimes our alleged strength becomes a double-edged sword as we are also told that we are too strong, too hard, too cold to deserve love, respect, and tenderness. "Black women are told that they are tough, pushy, and in charge rather than soft, feminine, and vulnerable. The image makes her someone to be feared (think Omarosa) rather than someone to be loved. These stereotypes render Black women as caricatures instead of whole people with strengths and weaknesses, tender sides and tough edges. And ultimately they make Black women invisible because they are not seen for all that they really are," write Charisse Jones and Dr. Kumea Shorter-Gooden in *Shifting—The Double Lives of Black Women in America.*

In one survey of black women, 67 percent agreed with the statement "Everyone expects me to be strong for them," and 47 percent agreed or strongly agreed with the statement "I am taking care of everyone else but no one is taking care of me." This is a common by-product of the SBW syndrome; people automatically assume you have the strength to get through, so nobody offers the consoling words because you appear to have it all under control. The truth is we do need our confidence boosted and our self-esteem refueled. We have difficulty stabilizing emotionally after a heartbreak, betrayal, or a personal or professional setback, just as anyone else does.

Our spiritual beliefs may also make us feel that suffering and self-sacrifice are part of the course of a Christian woman. After all, the course of God's people in the Bible is a story of a people led from one struggle to another. Many churches use scripture and sayings such as "God doesn't put more on you than you can bear," "What doesn't kill you will make you stronger," or "Weeping may endure for the night, buy joy cometh in the morning" to enforce an idea that suffering and self-sacrifice are ways to please God. Psychologists say that some women enjoy this form of self-punishment, which is akin to Christ's suffering in their mind. They can feel stronger, more powerful, from feeling a closer connection to God. To this, I would add the words of one ordained minister and professor of religion at a women's college: "There's a difference between being selfless and having no self at all." Developing a Christ-like attitude of putting others before yourself does not mean being a doormat for others to walk over.

How to Cope

1. Be strong, black, and a woman, but kick the whole Strong Black Woman supermyth to the curb. It's not realistic to be

there for everyone, handle every crisis, be the consummate professional, or require less from lovers than they do from you. As my girlfriend says, "There's a difference between a strong black woman and a strong black fool."

2. Draw strength from the remarkable legacy of black women, but use our power to rewrite our belief systems. Practice self-caretaking. When you take care of yourself, you can do more, love more, and, most importantly right now, improve your chances of bringing a healthy child into the world.

3. Repeat after me, "I am not Wonder Woman." Heck, even the real Wonder Woman only had to fight bad guys for thirty minutes every week, and she had her own personal jet, bulletproof bracelets, and a truth-telling rope. Find another way to deal with trials instead of internalizing them, convincing yourself that you can handle it. Write about it (throw it away afterward, if you want), talk about it, shout about it—just let it out.

4. Recognize your typical SBW responses. Recognizing it is the first step in releasing it. Practice saying, "No." Practice saying, "I can't."

WORK

Research by the Rollins School of Public Health at Emory University concluded that the racism experienced by black women in the workplace, both before and during pregnancy, is a key stressor that contributes to high-risk pregnancies and adverse birth outcomes.

Many of us are the only or one of few black women on the job, a situation increasingly known as "The Onlys." How can you really explain what it feels like to spend a greater part of your waking hours in a place where no one understands your perspective as black and female? For some reason we feel obligated to represent and defend the entire black race while performing our job duties. Consider the feelings of one woman in the Rollins School study:

I realize that anything I do on my job or out in public is going to impact how somebody else gets an impression about another black female. —JAMILIA, A WOMAN IN HER THIRTIES WORKING IN A CORPORATE SETTING

Sound familiar? It's bad enough to be the only one there, but then you have the ignorant comments, racist jokes, and innuendos. And you feel responsible for correcting every stereotype they've accepted as the gospel truth. I'll never forget when the only other black woman at work walked in with braids. The questions from ignorant white folks poured in like a final round of *Jeopardy!*, culminating with my two favorites—"Can you wash it?" and "Can I touch it?" I thought the poor sister was going to lose it on that last one.

Early in my career, I landed a job at a prominent national business magazine, where I was subjected to a racist supervisor. She would walk into my office with a resume and say, "Kimberly, does this name sound black to you?" That's a direct quote, by the way. She was engaged in one of those highly verbal—minimal results diversity campaigns, allegedly trying to add to the African American ranks. The current black roster stood at a whopping two, me included. She enlisted me in this farce, and I felt obligated to help, although diversity recruitment was not part of my job title and I was still expected to perform all of my usual duties. Once I busted her creating different hiring standards for the black candidates—insisting they should have, for example, three years of related work experience when there were plenty of white people who walked in straight out of college: no experience, no questions asked. The humdinger was when I confronted her about why after all this time, despite a stack of resumes from qualified black candidates, there had not been one hire. She said it was hard to find qualified black people and ended with, "Well, you know, Kimberly, you are only 13 percent of the population." Well, at this point, my Brooklyn instincts took over and I nearly jumped over the desk and attacked the old bag. Instead, I calmly walked out, went to my office, and drafted a memo to Human Resources.

When I had my sit-down with the powers that be, I revealed that one of the main sources of my anger and stress over the situation was that I was not allowed the luxury of going to work with just work on my mind. I had to strategize how I would avoid this woman or respond to her ignorant comments. And I had to research what kind of sedative I needed to be on, so as not to knock her out one day. What I really wanted was to go to the office and focus on work. It seems simple, but it was so unattainable for me for all those months that I suffered under that oppressive supervisor, figuring that I could handle it. I had landed this "good job" and didn't want to be viewed as a "complainer" or a "problem." During that time I was physically ill, fatigued, depressed, and riddled with ulcers. I am thankful I wasn't pregnant at the time. But these kinds of continued or episodic stresses can take their toll on the body, leaving it weaker later on during pregnancy. In fact, researchers are now increasingly studying lifetime stress, not just stress during pregnancy, as a factor in birth outcomes.

How to Cope:
1. Learn to let stuff roll off your back.
2. If you get an e-mail or memo that really sets you off, write a nasty reply, but don't press Send, says Dr. Angela Neal-Barnett, an award-winning psychologist and director of the Program for Research on Anxiety Disorders among African Americans at Kent State University. "Keeping your feelings in is not good for you or your baby. Allow yourself to vent. Then hold on to that response for a day, and then make a response (if needed) that's more appropriate."
3. Do not take on the role of the walking Black Encyclopedia or feel it's your job single-handedly to change all negative perceptions of black people. Repeat after me: "All I can do is be the best person I can be."
4. "Ignorance withers in the face of calm, confident intelligence," says Dr. Angela Neal-Barnett, author of *Soothe Your Nerves: A Black Woman's Guide to Understanding and Overcoming Anxiety,*

Panic and Fear. So the next time you get hit with an ignorant comment, don't go off. Consider other options such as the scathing look and walk-away response that allow you to keep your cool and get someplace else where you can vent, she suggests.

5. Pamper yourself. While aromatherapy can't relieve stress entirely, it can't hurt. "I like to add a half ounce of my favorite bath or sea salts to my foot bath. Then I add a tablespoon of olive oil and soak away for ten to fifteen minutes. The salts soften dry skin and calluses, and the olive oil moisturizes," suggests Sherri from Michigan. Or try this suggestion from Mya from New Orleans. "My favorite foot-bath recipe is to swish one and a half cups of cider vinegar and half a cup of fresh lemon juice in warm water."

RELATIONSHIPS

Relationships are stressful enough when you're not pregnant. But a pregnancy, particularly if unplanned, can put an extra strain on any relationship, married or not. Simone, a sassy fireplug (as my grandma would say) from Dayton, Ohio, was worried about how pregnancy and a baby would affect her relationship with her boyfriend. Would he find my new body attractive? Would he love me any less? she wondered. And although she had been in a committed relationship for five years, they were unmarried. "The stress of people trying to tell me what to do or giving me the dirty look because I was unmarried was too much," she says. She thought she was all right with their decision not to hurry their marriage plans, but the pressure mounted. At about six months into her pregnancy, Simone secretly bought a wedding band to wear on the appropriate finger when she went to the grocery store or other public places. She never told her man about the ring. Even worse, Simone never communicated with him about her changed feelings about getting married. "I didn't know how he would respond, and I was afraid that if the response wasn't what I wanted and needed it to be, it would be too much of a disappointment to handle," she says. That was Simone's cardinal emotional sin. The worse thing you can do is to keep any relationship anxiety to yourself. Dr. Neal-Barnett agrees. "Most of the time what you imagine will happen is much worse than what will actually happen," the good doctor says.

How to Cope:

1. If you have anxiety about your relationship, talk about it. Carve out forty-five minutes to an hour to sit down and talk without TV, telephone, or other interruptions.

2. When having a sensitive conversation about your relationship, Dr. Neal-Barnett suggests, start with, "This is how I am feeling," and then ask, "How are you feeling?" If your man is having difficulty expressing himself, be patient. Don't jump to a conclusion that he doesn't care. "Black men also have fears, insecurities and anxieties, but it's looked down upon for them to express these feelings," says Dr. Neal-Barnett. "Sadly, there are a lot of frightened black men on our streets."

3. Rejuvenate your faith in God and his ability to handle all matters. And rekindle your faith in yourself that no matter what happens, you will be able to handle it.

The Disease to Please

It is a known and undisputable fact that black women spend a lot of time taking care of others. Many of us are raised to believe that there is nothing more noble than giving up ourselves for others. When you are asked to do something, do you answer yes without considering the consequences to yourself? A young woman in Saint Louis found herself about seven months pregnant and on her hands and knees cleaning the house of an elderly woman she and her husband helped out on a regular basis. She knew she had no business doing that kind of work at that stage of her pregnancy.

She was tired and needed to rest, and she often felt ill after working at the woman's house. But she didn't know how to say no when
she received the call from the woman for help. She forgot that her
first responsibility was to her own health and well-being and that
of her baby. Remember, if you're not healthy, you can be of little
use to others.

If your sense of duty to others crosses the line and you can't turn
it off, the problem could be serious. Do you worry about what
people will think of you or fear being criticized by others? Dr.
Neal-Barnett calls it a disease to please and it falls under the category of social anxieties. Are you trying to please everyone, take care
of others, or lend money to relatives, all in the name of helping?
This sense of obligation is particularly stressful when you are pregnant, because taking care of yourself is extremely demanding on its
own. If your role as the go-to person in your family, the family
ATM machine, or the listening ear for everyone's drama is taxing
you, you need to take positive steps now.

How to Cope:

1. Practice saying no without feeling guilty. "Sometimes saying
   no, is the best thing you can do for someone because they
   learn to do for themselves," says Dr. Neal-Barnett. The more
   you practice it, the easier it becomes to say no.

2. Listen to your body. Become more aware of your limits and
   learn when you have reached them. Treat yourself more. Even
   an at-home pedicure or facial works. Try this: blend sea salts,
   blue cornmeal, and almond oil together for an invigorating
   foot scrub and soak.

3. "Practice the So What Chorus," says the doctor. So what, you
   said no. So what if so and so doesn't like you as much. So what
   that you chose to take care of yourself first this time.

4. Ask yourself, How would I feel or what would be accomplished if I pleased everyone else and ended up harming my
   baby? Is it really worth the risk?

HAVING IT ALL/DOING IT ALL

Sisters, we have a problem. We want it all—careers, husband, children, big house, two-car garage, the SUV, the works. The good news is that we've raised the bar as to what is attainable for us. And why not? We come from a long line of women who did it all even when they didn't have it all. And for the thirty- and forty-something generation we had our weekly icon—Clair Huxtable, Esq. Clair Huxtable showed a generation of future lawyers, doctors, and accountants that upwardly mobile black women could indeed have it all. We could raise five kids without a nanny, take care of a house, maintain a high-powered career, be adored by our husband, and still look glamorous and sexy. Though that was true, it is still TV. The bad news is that the pursuit of having it all is a tiring quest. It can weigh on us like a millstone—causing heaving burdens to our bodies and our spirits. The truth is that no one can do everything well. If you vigorously pursue all those aspects of having it all, you will not succeed at all of them. Something will fall through the cracks. The goal of having it all and doing it all is based on a myth, and trying to do it all during pregnancy is a recipe for trouble. My favorite advice in this regard is from CNN's Soledad O'Brien's: "Set a low bar." Hear more from Soledad on page 136. She was talking about during pregnancy and beyond. When you set realistic goals, you don't have the frustration and stress of not reaching impractical levels.

That also works with doing it all. I've met a lot of women who have their mama's high standards about having a clean and tidy house, or ironing clothes, and doing other housework. When you're trying to do the healthy meals, get your rest, keep up with the laundry, clean the house, and prepare for the baby, it can be a bit much. Don't be afraid to ask for or pay for help. Phyllis, from Chicago, was in a financial position to get some help with housework. But the idea that another person would clean her house was so foreign to her, so removed from her idea of what moms do, she never even considered it. When she heard about other moms who got household help, and another who had a personal chef prepare enough meals for the week, she started to investigate. When she realized that in her area, she could get two Russian women to clean her house for about sixty dollars a week, she was floored. She couldn't believe she was tiring herself and stressing out over a messy house when help was readily available.

And, yes, you may feel that nobody cleans your house the way you clean. This is likely true, but so what? Clean is clean. Try to do the things that you feel you absolutely must do and then delegate the others. Get your priorities straight. Finding time to rest, and to be alone with your thoughts, is more important than washing a basket of laundry. If you're like me, and you can't sleep knowing there are unwashed dishes in the kitchen or dirty clothes in the hamper, ask someone else to clean them or move them out of sight. And then go take a nap.

How to Cope:
1. Set realistic goals. Delegate.
2. Lose the perfectionist tendencies. A lot of us subscribe to the old adage "If you want something done right, you have to do it yourself." But what you really mean is that if you want something done *your way*, then you have to do it yourself. To delegate you need to accept that "my way" of doing things is not the only effective one. You will learn that things will get done when they need to get done, even if it's not on your timetable.
3. Get help. Research the costs of a monthly or biweekly cleaner/ maid service. A responsible teenager can also wash dishes, mop the floor, or fold laundry and may work for even less money.

Let It Go
Five Ways to De-stress

If bubble baths and scented candles aren't really working for you, here are some other ideas to reduce stressful feelings and regain a peaceful center:

Count Your Blessings: The more you focus on life's problems, the more stressed out you feel. You'll feel better by asking yourself what is right with your life. Make a list or keep an Appreciation Journal. You may realize that it's pretty hard to be in an appreciative state and a stressed-out state at the same time. Making a list gives you something to refer to when things are difficult or stressful. Some ideas to add to your appreciation journal:

The feeling of joy after lending a helping hand
Acknowledgment you received from a boss, friend, or loved one
Something you did for someone else that gave her joy
Your valued talents and qualities
Hearing the laughter of a child
Your accomplishments in life

Practice Deep Breathing: When you're stressed, you have a tendency to breathe more shallowly and rapidly, which deprives your body of vital oxygen. To prompt a relaxation response, try to reverse the pattern by breathing slowly and deeply. Breathe from the abdomen instead of the chest. Take a deep breath from your abdomen, count to 4 in your mind, and exhale until the count of 8. Do this several times, and you can instantly release pressure and shift your focus away from your emotions to the breath.

Rearrange or Redecorate Your Environment: Either in an office, in a cubicle or at home, your surroundings can be soothing or comforting or jarring, annoying, or painful. Color, lighting, and sound are all elements that engage and influence the senses. Light therapy has been proven to help treat migraines, premenstrual syndrome (PMS), some cancers, and other diseases. The idea of light therapy isn't new. The connection between light and health and vitality was very strong in ancient times. And I'm sure your mama always told you to go outside and get some fresh air and sunshine. She wasn't just trying to get you out of her hair—or maybe she was. But it was good for you just the same. The sounds around us can also ease or increase stress. Become aware of how noise affects you and what you can do about it. And color is known to have emotional and physiological benefits.

Affirmations: Find some pick-me-up phrases that work for you and post these notes in places you'll see them often, like your computer monitor, car visor, bathroom mirror, or refrigerator door. Try sayings like "Don't sweat the small stuff" or "I love and accept myself as I am." These can help boost your self-confidence and reduce stress, too. Try a book like *Black Pearls: Daily Meditations, Affirmations and Inspirations for African Americans* by Eric V. Copage. In fact, instead of waiting until you're stressed out to refer to an affirmation, begin the day with your saying or another inspirational text that lifts your spirit and sets a peaceful tone for the day.

Do Something for Someone Else: Take a moment to smile at a stranger, send a just-because "e-card," hold the door for someone. You'll feel calmer and create an energy that opens you up to the kindness of others and puts you in good stead to reap what you have sown.

Keep Your Cool
Four Ways to Defuse Drama

*N*obody can work a nerve the way a friend, a relative, or even your husband can, when you're pregnant. Try these suggestions:

Get off the Phone Gently When a Conversation Gets Overheated. Tell the person that you want to address this issue/problem later, after you both have calmed down. If someone won't let you off the hook that easily, use one of many pregnancy excuses—you have to pee, go eat, throw up, call your doctor, or do all of the above.

Set Boundaries. Arin, a thirty-two-year old Ph.D. from Chicago, had a problem with her mother-in-law when she was pregnant. Her mother-in-law disapproved of Arin's high-powered career and work schedule. "It got to the point where she was mean and attacking me, saying things like 'Why are you working?' and 'What kind of mother will you be if you're working?' " Other times, her mother-in-law would call and talk ad infinitum about her own life problems. "I don't have time for her to go on and on. I would say, 'I understand you're upset, but what would you like me to do?' She thought I was being disrespectful." Matters reached a breaking point for Arin when after another heated discussion about work her mother-in-law said something that ended with "I don't care what happens to you."

"Around the sixth month of my pregnancy, I realized it is not my job to take care of her. I wrote down my priorities, of which the health of our baby and me was at the top," Arin says. "I confronted my husband and after a few knock-down-drag-out fights, we agreed that being stressed during this pregnancy and beyond is not an option for me. I asked him, 'Are you willing to put our child at risk over this situation?' " At that point, Arin set boundaries to keep her mental and emotional health intact. If she sees her mother-in-law's phone number on the caller ID, she lets it go to voice mail. She does not stay at her mother-in-law's house, and her mother-in-law does not stay at her home. "We've stuck to those rules. I had to have a space where I'm comfortable and relaxed. Besides, I don't want to raise my daughter to take crap from people. How can I teach her that if I'm not setting a good example?" Arin says.

Take Your Pick: Acute Pain or Chronic Pain. Here's a thought that I know Arin applied in her situation: would you rather deal with acute pain, which can be momentarily sharp and then go away, or chronic pain that lingers forever? You can confront the problem, deal with the high drama that may last days or weeks, or you can let a situation cause you pain, possibly for the rest of your life. Remember: there is no such thing as a diplomatic hand grenade. Choosing not to deliver a difficult message is like hanging on to a hand grenade once you've pulled the pin. It is better to deal with it and be done.

Express Your Need. Your choice of words can either deffuse or escalate a situation. Using the word *need* makes the person on the other end feel special and important in your life. It also makes him or her involved in your well-being. "I really need you to talk to someone else on this one because I am . . ." or "I really need you to stop doing/saying this because it makes me feel. . . ."

ReTell Therapy

A MOTHERLESS CHILD,
PREGNANCY AFTER THE LOSS OF MY MOM

by Karen Shaw

It was 4:30 A.M. on Friday, May 9. The telephone rang. I jumped up out of the bed to answer it, sensing it was bad news. "Karen, I am not getting any breath," the voice said. It was my mother's caretaker. "Okay," I said. "I will be right there." I quickly woke up my husband and said, "Let's go; Mommy is gone." This was the moment I always dreaded—my mother's death. Since the age of six or seven I would have terrible daydreams that my mother would leave me. That day arrived. And it was one of the saddest days in my life.

About one month after my mother's death I found out that I was pregnant with my second child. As I looked up from the pregnancy test, I realized that I conceived the week of my mother's funeral. Now instead of diving into a hectic work routine to help forget the pain of losing my best friend, I was pregnant again, but this time without my mother! And so soon. What would I do? My mother, my rock, my confidante, and rhythm to my beat was not here to guide me.

I was still grieving and physically and emotionally exhausted from my mother's prolonged illness. I began to evaluate my life and create a survival plan for raising a family without any family of my own to help me. My mother and I were both only children, and I had very little contact with my father after my parents' divorce when I was age two. How could I raise children, maintain a career and my marriage, without my mother's help and support? Somehow, I had to heal and move on. After all, I did get pregnant the week of her funeral, proving that life continues.

I thought about my life. Armed with my M.B.A. I was another

black woman trying to pierce the corporate glass ceiling. I lived a high-stress lifestyle, made bad food choices, got little rest, and pushed myself until I passed out from exhaustion.

My health became the most important thing. Through my mother's illness I learned that too much stress is not good. My mother worked hard and rarely relaxed. I often felt that this caused her illness. Without my mother as my stress reliever, I knew I had to make drastic changes. I decided not to go back to stressful corporate America, but to stay at home with my children and start an at-home business. While the six-figure salary was very attractive, I valued my sanity and peace of mind much more.

Holistic and alternative medicine had always been a strong interest of mine. For years, I advised people on how to heal themselves through herbs and natural remedies. I found a multilevel marketing business that was a perfect fit. I also enrolled in a Ph.D. holistic nutrition class to further my knowledge of the field.

In addition to giving out health advice, I became my best customer and designed a prenatal herbal program. The diet change and herbs gave me lots of energy, no swelling, and a great outlook on the new life inside me. I took yoga classes and had monthly massages. Next, I designed a support network. I found Mocha Moms, a group of black stay-at-home moms. New friends can't replace my mother, but I realized that family is what you make it.

My pregnancy journey without my mother was truly a life changing experience. While not physically here to assist with the everyday rituals of motherhood, her spirit helped me redefine myself and set new goals for my family.

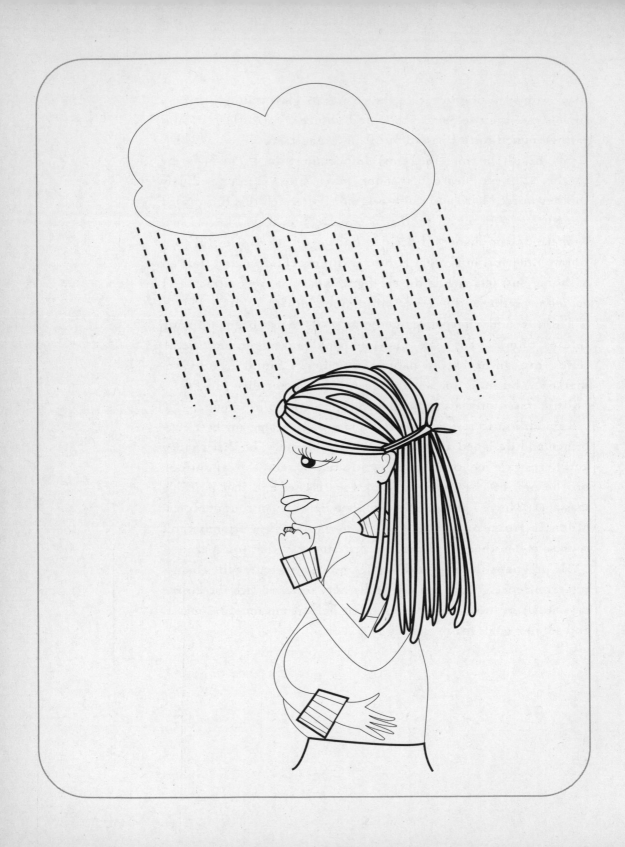

8

The Darker Side of Pregnancy

Depression, Loss, and Postabortion Support

Despite all of the radiant glowing and happiness that society associates with pregnancy, for many women this is not the case at all. The glossy pregnancy magazines and all the smiling, content faces, filled with euphoric expectation and boundless joy, do not represent everyone's pregnancy experience. Instead of feelings of happiness, many women feel confusion, fear, sadness, stress, and even depression. Others start off on the happy journey, but a miscarriage or other loss leaves them shocked and in pain.

Depression

About 10 to 20 percent of women will struggle with symptoms of depression during pregnancy, and a quarter to half of these will suffer from major depression. It is not that surprising a condition when you consider that pregnancy depression is a mood disorder just as normal depression is. Mood disorders are biological illnesses that involve changes in brain chemicals. And since pregnancy hormones can affect brain chemicals directly related to depression and anxiety, pregnant women can be, in some cases, more susceptible.

The bigger problem with depression as it relates to black women is that symptoms closely resemble something we call life. We have convinced ourselves that feeling sad, overwhelmed, lonely, and sick and tired are part and parcel of being a black woman, particularly a strong black woman. So we have a lot of denial about depression, which our folk negatively label as being "crazy," "weak," or "lazy." We rationalize that being a strong black woman, from a line of similar women who survived with an indomitable spirit, somehow makes us immune to depression. The statistics on black women are scarce and uncertain, not because we don't suffer from depression but because we don't associate those types of feelings with a real illness, but rather with a passing phase that we shall overcome. We have misguided beliefs about our ability to persevere. I mean, c'mon, we've been through slavery, Reconstruction, segregation, Jim Crow, Reaganomics, and we're still kickin', we reason. And when we consider what our parents, grandparents, and great-grandparents went through (and they will remind us!), we figure they've had it much worse so we best shut up and "deal with it." We got Jesus, Oprah, and now, Dr. Phil, so somehow we'll make it through.

Yet, African American women report depression symptoms including restlessness, boredom, and anxiety more than black men and white women and men. We also have a depression rate that is two times higher than that of European American women, according to one study. Other research puts that depression rate at three times higher than white women's.

It's no wonder when you consider the triple-whammy, high-risk status of most black women. "We live in a majority-dominated society that frequently devalues our ethnicity, culture, and gender. Often we are involved in multiple roles as we attempt to survive economically and advance ourselves and our families through mainstream society. All of these factors intensify the amount of stress within our lives which can erode our self-esteem, social support systems, and health," writes Barbara Jones Warren, a psychiatric mental health nurse consultant and professor at Ohio State University in a research paper.

"We are innovators who have historically have been involved in the development of family and group survival strategies. However, women may experience increased stress, guilt and depressive symptoms when they have role conflicts between their family's survival and their own developmental needs. It is this cumulative stress which takes a toll on the strengths of African-American women and can produce an erosion of emotional and physical health," continues Jones Warren. Looking after everyone else will invariably lead to neglecting yourself.

We feel hurt or depressed, but we just don't call it depression. We call it "the blues," "a funk," or "a little down." The National Mental Health Association says that only two-thirds of those with depression receive treatment. In black communities, "the percentage of people with symptoms that go unrecognized or misdiagnosed is even higher," according to the Association.

The biggest problem with depression during pregnancy is that some of the symptoms of depression—fatigue, weight change, and anxiety—are very similar to the side effects of pregnancy. Women who have depression also usually experience at least three of the following symptoms for two weeks or more:

* A depressed, irritable, or sad mood throughout the day (often every day)
* Difficulty in concentrating
* Too much or too little sleep
* Loss of interest in activities you usually enjoy
* Recurring thoughts of death, suicide, or hopelessness
* Anxiety
* Unusual, agitated, or decreased physical activity (generally every day)

* Feelings of guilt or worthlessness
* Change in eating habits/eating too much or too little
* Significant weight loss or gain (more than 5 percent) over one
  month

Society's perceptions of a happy pregnancy can propel you deeper into feelings of guilt and anxiety. Barbara, from Bowie, Maryland, found her pregnancy depression particularly confusing because she wanted to be pregnant. She and her husband tried for over a year before she was able to conceive. "I couldn't figure out why I felt so bad when everyone, including myself, expected me to feel so good." After a lot of investigation, Barbara's mother reluctantly admitted she, too, suffered with depression throughout her life, as had Barbara's grandmother. Barbara was shocked to find this "secret" lurking in her family history, and unbeknownst to her, this history of depression made her at a higher risk for development of pregnancy depression.

Poverty, the loss of a loved one, job-related frustrations or other life traumas are also a possible trigger. Other risks include the following:

* Age at the time of pregnancy: the younger you are, the higher
  the risk.
* A personal prepregnancy history of depression.
* Living alone.
* Limited social support.
* Chronic or serious illnesses. (Some doctors believe that people
  who have chronic illnesses—cancer, heart disease, diabetes, and
  the like—have bodies that are prone to development of other
  illness: that there is an actual change in the physiology of the
  person that actually leads to the development of depression.)
* Marital conflict.
* Ambivalence about the pregnancy.
* History of abuse or trauma.
* Previous pregnancy loss.

Depression can have several negative effects on your pregnancy and baby. Studies have shown that babies born to depressed mothers have lower birth weight, higher risk of premature birth and birth complications, delayed cognitive and language development, and more behavioral problems (sounds as if your mama's warning that "If you're sad, your baby will be sad," isn't just an old wive's tale). Scientists figure that there's something about the unbalanced sea of hormones and reduced blood flow that these babies are exposed to in the womb that causes these effects.

Other damage can be seen even before the baby is born. Depression usually interferes with a woman's ability to take care of herself during pregnancy. You may be less likely to follow all the medical recommendations or to sleep and eat properly. The risk of using substances like tobacco, alcohol, and legal and illegal drugs, which can harm a growing fetus, increases with depression. And depression may interfere with your ability to bond with your growing baby. It is medically proven that a baby can recognize the mother's voice and sense emotion by pitch, rhythm, and stress while in the womb. Pregnant women who have depression find it more difficult to develop this bond and feel more detached and emotionally isolated from the pregnancy experience. Also, pregnancy depression puts you at a higher risk for postpartum depression.

The prevalence of, and issues related to, pregnancy depression are so serious researchers are now devoting more efforts to its study. A team of doctors at the University of Michigan Depression Center Women's Mood Disorders Program conducted a survey over a three-year period at a variety of clinics where pregnant women were awaiting their prenatal doctor's visits. The women ranged in age from ten to forty-six years old, with an average age of 28.6, and had different racial and ethnic backgrounds, about 73 percent were white. They were on average about twenty-five weeks into their pregnancies. The survey used a questionnaire about current distress and depressive feelings, alcohol use, lifetime and recent depression history and treatment, overall health, use of prescription drugs, and demographic characteristics. They were also asked whether they had had a period of two or more weeks in the last six months, or in their lifetime, when they had consistently felt sad, blue, or depressed or had lost all interest in things such as work—an indication of major depression. The result: 28 percent of the women said they had a lifetime history of major depression, and 42 percent scored high enough to indicate that they were currently experiencing minor or major depression.

If pregnancy depression is so rampant, why aren't more people talking about it? Pregnancy books devote small, scattered paragraphs to the subject. Everyone has a Kool-Aid grin in the magazines. Even the pregnancy bible, *What to Expect When You're Expecting*, devotes less than one full page to the topic. "There's a lot of stuff on postpartum depression. I guess, to be depressed after birth is more socially accepted and understood, but being depressed during pregnancy is a different story," says Carlise of Maywood, Illinois.

What to Do

* If you're depressed, take off the strong black woman superhero outfit. Pack it away. If your belief system says, I'm strong and should be able to handle all situations, when the occasion inevitably arises that you can't do these things, you think you're a failure. Those feelings can lead to depression.

* Listen to this anecdote from the psychiatric nurse consultant Jones Warren: "I remember one of my clients, a woman who had been brought into the emergency mental health center because she had slashed her wrists while at work. During my assessment of her, she told me she felt like she was 'dragging a weight around all the time.' She said, 'I've had all these tests done and they tell me physically everything is fine but I know it's not. Maybe I'm going crazy! Something is terribly wrong with me, but I don't have time for it. I've got a family who depends on me to be strong. I'm the one that everyone turns to.' This woman, more concerned about her family than her-

self, said she '[felt] guilty spending so much time on [her]self.' When I asked her if she had anyone she could talk to, she responded, 'I don't want to bother my family and my closest friend is having her own problems right now.' Her comments reflect and mirror the sentiments of other depressed African-American women I have seen in my practice: They're alive, but barely, and are continually tired, lonely, and wanting."

✳ Recognize that pregnancy depression is very serious. Not seeking help is putting your baby in danger. You have a baby inside you who needs you to be physically, emotionally, and mentally healthy. Again, I will repeat what I have said is one of the best gems of pregnancy advice I've heard throughout my journey with this book. Soledad O'Brien told me that her doctor simply stated, "You can put in the time on the front end, taking care of yourself, or you will put in the time on the back end, when you spend your days and nights in an NICU [neonatal intensive care unit] trying to nurse a sickly baby back to health. But either way, you will put in the time."

✳ Can you lighten your load? Cut down on your chores, errands for others, and other stressful activities. Try to do things that will help you relax and regroup.

✳ If your trigger is relationship related, remember that if a relationship goes bad, it doesn't mean that we've failed or that we can't ever have a fulfilling relationship. It just means that particular relationship didn't work out for us. You cannot hold yourself responsible for another person's choice. Surround yourself with positive stories of successful single mothers, couples who've drastically improved their marital situation, and women who have thrived after freeing themselves from abusive relationships.

✳ Talk. As simple as this may sound, black people are socialized not to air dirty laundry, so to speak. We are reluctant to share our problems, particularly with strangers. Talk to your doctor, a friend, a trusted relative. If you feel embarrassed, call an anonymous hotline or your employer's Employee Assistance

Program, if available. Never try to face depression alone when you are pregnant; your baby needs you to seek help.

✳ Find support groups. Group sessions can be more supportive for many women, providing a place to help understand depression and what can be done about it. And most of all, there is often comfort in numbers. Knowing, and actually seeing, that you are not alone is sometimes the powerful tool for overcoming negative feelings. Contact the National Black Women's Health Project for information on some of its support groups (see Appendix).

✳ Consider private therapy. Choose a culturally competent professional who understands the complexities of a black woman's life (see Appendix). Studies prove that we are more likely to receive better treatment and respond to it when we have such a therapist. Some black therapists recommend a complete medical and family history and cultural assessment to help determine the root cause of the depression.

✳ Be open to other therapies, including light, meditation, and relaxation therapy; programs that help you develop alternate crisis management and coping skills; and programs for improving nutrition and exercise.

✳ Medication may help. Sometimes depression can be extreme. There are no triggers, no known causes. If you won the lottery tomorrow, you would still be sad. If your symptoms are severe, your doctor may suggest some medication. A warning: studies show that black women may be more sensitive to certain antidepressants and may require smaller dosages than usually prescribed. So do your research on the different types of medications and their effects.

OOPS! DEALING WITH UNINTENDED PREGNANCIES

According to the National Survey of Family Growth, 49 percent of all pregnancies in the United States (excluding miscarriages) and

31 percent of all pregnancies resulting in live births are unintended. If you are struggling to accept an unplanned pregnancy, the greatest comfort may just be knowing that you are not alone. Twenty-eight percent of women have had at least one unplanned birth. For a woman, an unplanned pregnancy can be the source of great stress, and sometimes of negative feelings.

Black women can have more initial adverse reactions to unintended pregnancies because we tend to have stronger control issues. We have a tough time dealing with things that "aren't supposed to happen." We could easily beat ourselves up, thinking, "How could this happen?" and end up mired in guilt. The truth is, unplanned pregnancies happen—and quite often, that is, according to the stats. In state-by-state data collected by the Centers for Disease Control, the percentages of black women giving birth after unplanned pregnancies in various states ranged from 46.2 to 76.7 percent. Not surprisingly, Colorado was the state with the lowest incidence of such pregnancies (presumably because it has a low incidence of spotting an actual black person anyway). And Illinois was the state with highest prevalence (let's hear it for Chi-Town!). Let's face it, condoms break, the pill does fail, a heated moment of passion leaves your birth control on the floor with your panties instead of where it is supposed to be, and we have all heard about a woman who got pregnant even though her tubes were tied!

By the government's definition, an unintended pregnancy is either mistimed (the woman wanted to be pregnant later) or unwanted (she did not want ever to be pregnant). There is an interest in these data because they may affect a woman's behavior and experiences during the pregnancy and affect the health of the baby.

Specifically, women who have mistimed pregnancies are likely to discover their pregnancies later than those who have planned pregnancies, and that makes them less likely to get an early start with prenatal care. You may already know how important folic acid is in the early, early stages of pregnancy in the prevention of neural tube defects. In fact, if you are planning on getting pregnant your doctor will likely tell you to beef up the folic acid months before conception. Unplanned or unwanted pregnancies can also affect infant health, since studies show that women who have unintended births are less likely to breast-feed, and breast-fed babies have fewer respiratory and ear infections and have been proven to have a higher IQ.

Most of the women I met worried that the timing was just *wrong*—their husband had recently lost his job, they'd just moved, they were having marital or other relationship issues, their career was just taking off, or they were on the cusp of an overdue promotion. Others, who already had children, just considered themselves "done" and put the thoughts of crying babies, late night feedings, and diaper Genies, completely out of their mind (read Jeanne Whitfield's ReTell Therapy on page 210). But as my husband often says, "If the world only had babies who came just at the right time, there wouldn't be many of them on the planet." If you ask around your family, you may be shocked at how many "surprises" there are in your group; you may also find that even you were an "unexpected blessing," as my mother would say.

A lot of your anxiety may be centered around your spouse's or partner's response. He may not be very excited about the idea. A man's anxiety about fatherhood often stems from financial concerns and worries over how he will provide. He may even blame you. "I was reaching for the condom, and *you* said don't worry about it." Do not let him play the blame game. It still takes two to make a baby, so there is a shared responsibility. Do not feel you let him down or you betrayed his trust in you. Take responsibility for your actions and ask him to do the same, remembering that pointing fingers and wallowing in guilt are not going to change anything.

Dianne, married only three months when she became pregnant, struggled to feel good about her pregnancy. Even though her husband was happy and supportive, she couldn't help but feel secretly saddened. In fact, his excitement made her feel more guilty and upset. "We just got married. After investing so much time into finding a life partner, I couldn't believe that my plans for how I envisioned married life were ruined. We wanted to travel, live abroad, and drive cross country," she says. "We had a small apartment and were financially recovering from an expensive wedding and honeymoon. I just couldn't believe it." She faked excitement to her friends and family, but she spent most of her time alone in tears.

It took several months for Dianne to get over her negative thoughts. She forced herself to eat healthy meals, but "I was motivated by duty—nothing more," she says. She really turned the corner when her belly swelled and ultimately when she got her first little kick. "That's when it really hit me. Literally. I just woke up the next day and said I was going to stop whining about what didn't go right and focus on my baby. I made a conscious effort to be positive." You can do the same.

What to Do

* Think positive. Negative feelings can be so overwhelming we forget that we have options. We can wrongly assume that the present situation is the cause; therefore, the only option is to ride out the problem to the end. But you can choose to respond and react differently. You have the option to make a change for yourself. The next time you're feeling negative thoughts, stop yourself and ask, Can I respond differently this time? How can I adjust my thinking?

* Propagandize yourself. Immerse yourself in the wonderful world of maternity and motherhood. Get the magazines, buy more books—soak up all the positive information about pregnancy you can find.

* Be honest. Don't give yourself the extra burden of keeping up a pretense of happiness. You are not the first person to have ambivalent or negative feelings about pregnancy. Try, "It's an adjustment, but I'm getting there."

* Do something. When you start to feel sad, go for a stroll through a local baby store, Ooohing over the cute outfits you'll be buying soon. If it works with your budget, buy a small item,

maybe booties or a bib. Check out the strollers and other baby gear—it's never too late to start thinking about your gift registry.

✳ Count your blessings. Think of the millions of women out there who are desperately trying to have babies. They spend thousands of dollars on fertility treatments or fly across the world in search of a baby they can call their own—consider yourself blessed simply to have conceived.

✳ Have faith in yourself and God that you will make it through.

✳ Don't let people get to you. Inevitably, some insensitive friend or relative will make a comment like "However will you manage?" If you have a particular family member or friend who keeps going there, just say it's a topic that is not open for discussion—and then never talk about it again. And never be afraid to tell anybody who needs to be told, to mind his or her own business.

✳ Get help. If your feelings toward the pregnancy prevent you from taking care of yourself—eating properly, seeing your doctor, and soon—or linger into your second trimester, then you need to talk to a professional immediately.

You won't feel this way for long. Even if you think you have the maternal instincts of Mommy Dearest, you'll be surprised how actual motherhood will turn the staunchest of former antimotherhood crusaders into blubbering moms complete with teddy bear diaper bags and two brag books.

Pregnancy After an Abortion

There are a number of studies on how abortion affects a woman's later pregnancy experiences, and the results show that a great many women experience painful unresolved issues or postabortion grief during pregnancy. Did you know that 44 percent of all American women will have an abortion at some point during their lifetime? More than a million American women will have an abortion in any given year, but very few of them talk about it. Why is that?

For black women, abortion has historically been one of those things we label as something "white people do." A study by the *Los Angeles Times* in 2001 found that 56 percent of African Americans oppose most abortions compared to 54 percent of whites. But the startling statistics about black women and abortion reveal quite a different picture: white women obtain 58 percent of all abortions, but their abortion rate is well below that of African American women. Black women are more than three times as likely as white women to have an abortion. While only 14 percent of the women in the United States of childbearing age are African American, the most recent available statistics show that 35.9 percent of all abortions are performed on black women. In one of the more surprising findings, married black women have an abortion rate almost five times higher than that of married white women—this could indicate that either increased career opportunities or lack of job stability is affecting our choices about when and whether we become mothers.

Clearly, this is another taboo area in the black community. Let's face it: for years black families have dealt with out-of-wedlock children by just absorbing them into our larger family. As my grandmother would say, "We can always make room for one more mouth at the table."

Women who choose abortion are often, on some level, going against their own moral code, and this is why they feel guilt afterward. It is a rare woman who can truly go through the process, put the incident behind her, and get on with life as usual. You may try to forget but just can't. Even though we historically have a strong reliance on God and his boundless willingness to forgive, many women I interviewed spoke of a "What if?" type of lingering feeling. Residual feelings of guilt prevent hundreds of women from talking about it or getting the emotional help they need and deserve. For a number of sisters, it's just one more thing to "get over" and "keep it moving."

Doctors have now been able to identify a condition they call *postabortion syndrome* (PAS), which is defined as an ongoing inability to:

* Process and deal with the painful thoughts and emotions—especially guilt, anger, and grief—that result from one or more unplanned pregnancies and subsequent abortions
* Identify (much less grieve) the loss that has been experienced
* Feel at peace with God, herself, and others involved in the pregnancy and abortion decision

Without proper grieving, unaddressed feelings can be neatly tucked away for years, only to resurface during another pregnancy, especially given the emotional ups and downs of pregnancy. These feelings can be exacerbated and overwhelming when the abortion was a secret and you feel you can't explain your true feelings to anyone. The anxiety ranges from an irrational fear that God may somehow punish you in this pregnancy for the previous abortion to feelings of unworthiness as a mother because of a past decision.

A study of the relationship between abortion and later pregnancies and children published in the *Pre- and Perinatal Psychology Journal* revealed these comments:

> When I finally decided to have a baby, my abortion began to bother me. I had some difficulties with bleeding and premature labor. I was fearful that I would never be able to have children. Emotionally I was a wreck. I stayed in the bed for nearly six months of the pregnancy. . . . I was so anxious and fearful, and underneath was a ton of guilt. I cried all the time. I got sick of people telling me to "calm down" and "relax." They had no idea about my abortion. I realize that's why I was so upset all the time. —MEREDITH, A STUDY PARTICIPANT

The thought of bringing a child into the world can stir up guilt, anger, and depression over the child you have lost. Some women report pregnancies full of moments of bargaining with God not to punish them with a defective child.

> After my abortion, my pregnancies have been times of fear and anxiety. I kept expecting God was going to punish me with a retarded child because I

*had an abortion. I was always depressed and worried. When my daughter
was born, I felt like I didn't deserve to be a mother.* —CINDA, A STUDY
PARTICIPANT

Even though you are pregnant, you may view yourself as unworthy because of your past decision. Psychologists say abortion can damage your image of yourself and raise questions in your mind about your ability to be a good mother.

The bottom line is that unresolved issues about a past abortion can steal your joy while you are expecting this one. It can result in more anxiety during labor, and therefore increased difficulty in labor, which may contribute to a higher incidence of complications of delivery. The mother-child bonding experience can also be complicated by past trauma.

Mothers who have such unresolved feelings are known to be extremely overprotective and to be extreme spoilers, who give in to their child's every demand, all in an effort to alleviate feelings of guilt and failure.

What to Do

* Remember the pain. In order to heal you have to tear away the callus you've built up by denying and repressing painful emotions. Get help.

* If you hold any spiritual beliefs, then true healing may not occur until you feel reconciled with God. Talk to a spiritual adviser or an anonymous help hotline related to your particular faith (see Appendix).

* Release any anger about your decision.

* The need to grieve an aborted pregnancy is basically unheard of because it begs the question of how you grieve over something you willingly destroyed. But grieving is part of the healing process. Contact a postabortion help center (see Appendix).

PREGNANCY LOSS

There are few events as painful as losing a baby. All of the exciting feelings and happy expectations about pregnancy come to a screeching halt, and instead of celebrating a life, you are grieving over a death.

When most people think of pregnancy loss, the first thought is of miscarriage. But miscarriage is only one type of loss. Ectopic pregnancy, stillbirth, and neonatal death are in the same category and equally devastating. Unfortunately pregnancy loss is a common event; about one in five women will suffer pregnancy loss. Painfully, some women go through a labor that ends with the delivery of a stillborn baby (read Lela Rochon's account on page 214 and Phyllis Baldwin's story on page 212) or a disabled or sickly baby who dies days later. Even an early miscarriage can cause distress.

When a woman loses a baby, at any stage, there is profound sadness, loss, and a sense of failure. It can cause you to lose faith in your body and its ability to function properly. Many women are overwhelmed by concerns that they did something wrong or somehow caused the loss. You can spend countless hours replaying your every move, wondering whether it was that bag of groceries you carried, or the argument you had, or that flight of stairs you took, a trip or fall, or stress—but none of these has been proven to cause miscarriage.

Tamisha, a legal secretary from Long Beach, California, had what would be called a textbook pregnancy. She ate well, she exercised, and she and her husband were happily expecting the arrival of their firstborn. But four hours after the birth of her baby girl, the baby died as a result of some internal malformation that was not detected by ultrasound. "We were utterly and completely devastated," she says. At the hospital, the doctors and nurses avoided her, ignored her questions, or gave evasive answers. They said things like "Don't worry; you'll get over it" or "You're young; you'll have another baby." Considering that a hospital staff consists of medically trained individuals, it's surprising how many women felt this type of response only worsened their grief. "From the beginning, it was like, this is something not to be discussed," Tamisha now a mother of two, says. So many women would have preferred answers, instead of silence. If you have suffered a loss, you may have received similar treatment at the hospital.

With no real answers to fill the gaping void that now existed, Tamisha and her husband left the hospital with empty hands and empty hearts. Well-meaning friends and loved ones got rid of all the baby stuff that was in the house before she got home. "People acted like my baby didn't exist. My husband didn't want to talk about it. Nobody talked about it. People avoided eye contact with me. And when I did try to talk about it, people quickly changed the subject or left the room," she says.

Her grief was intensified by isolation as friends, family, and even her husband withdrew. "It was like, nobody really called me because they didn't know what to say. My friends with babies avoided me because they thought being around their babies would upset me. If there was anything where a baby might be around—a family dinner, baby shower, graduation party—I usually wasn't invited. Instead of helping, it just made me feel all alone in my mourning," she says. "They didn't understand that I didn't want to forget. I didn't want to get over it. I wanted to feel, and hurt, and grieve, and miss my baby."

Inevitably someone will make an insensitive comment. Someone may say that because you never "really knew" your baby, it is not that bad. Or that it is better this way—meaning a child dies before you've come to know her personality or really gotten to know her. *These people are utterly ignorant!!* We mothers know that we form an amazing bond in utero that makes the baby an active, breathing-human being to us. We sisters know our baby's personality way before it is born—from the way it kicks at 2:00 A.M. to the foods it makes us crave. But when you lose a baby late in your pregnancy or shortly after delivery, you are the only one who experienced this connection. Even your husband or partner may not get it.

Erica, a writer in New York City, had a typical pregnancy until

HELLP syndrome developed at twenty-four weeks. HELLP stands for *hemolysis* or rupture of the red blood cells, *elevated liver* enzyme levels in the blood, and *low* blood levels of *platelets*. HELLP is similar to preeclampsia, toxemia, and pregnancy-induced hypertension and the terms are often used interchangeably. Erica's blood pressure climbed to over 240/110, her kidneys failed, and she had an emergency C-section. Her baby, named Grace, lived three days before she died. The day started fairly normally for Erica as she headed to a work meeting in midtown Manhattan.

I didn't feel too good. But I thought it was something that I ate. I went to the bathroom, but nothing happened. I began to feel worse and I thought, something is not right. I went outside to catch a cab to the hospital but because of the rain and the heavy traffic the trip took nearly an hour. During the time in that cab, I went from discomfort to pain to continuous pain to the point where I was crying. I felt like something was really going wrong. When I finally got to the hospital, there was a lot of protein in my urine, and my blood pressure was rising. The doctor said I had the symptoms of HELLP syndrome and I was given two steroid injections to help mature the baby's lungs so we could make it to twenty-seven weeks. To them, twenty-seven weeks was the magic number for my baby's chance of survival. I was in some sort of Twilight Zone. I had heard about things like preeclampsia and HELLP syndrome but that was in the back of the pregnancy books and I hadn't gotten that far yet. Things got progressively worse, and during the night while I was sleeping the doctor came and said that they were going to have to take the baby right now. My kidneys had shut down, and my blood platelets were low. They had a perinatologist come in and explain to me the prognosis for a twenty-four-week-old fetus. I would not wish an emergency C-section on my worst enemy. All of a sudden the mood in the room changed. There were what seemed like hundreds of people in this frenetic energy and you know it's all for you. They had a priest come in and give me the Sacrament of the Sick, which is something they do if they think you might not make it. I realized that I was really, really ill. I sensed that at twenty-four weeks, they didn't expect the baby to live, but what was now clear was that they weren't sure if I was going to live. I heard them yell 200/110. Now, I'm not a doctor, but I know that is too high to be anybody's blood pressure. By this point, I'm crying and thinking, this might be it. You get to a point where you can choose to fear death, but if it's going to come, it's going to come. And so I had to say, Wow, this might be it. A priest came and prayed over me, for me, and with me. He absolved me of my sins. And I told them that I wanted to donate my organs. I'm lying there on an operating table and the only thing I can think about is, if I die will I go to heaven? When it was time for the anesthesia, he told me to count to ten. I remember counting to three and that was it. When I woke up, the first thing I heard was "She's alive, Erica." It was my partner, Kevin. She had been baptized, and he saw it. He said he heard her cry. It was amazing. She was under one pound. They wouldn't let me go see her. They said I was too ill. My pressure had gone up to 240 before they were able to stabilize me. That was very tough. How can you say that to a mother? Part of my recovery was to see her. When I did see her, it blew me away, she was so small, yet so perfect. This was the baby I was carrying. Over the next few days, I vacillated between wanting to see her so much and not wanting to see her at all because there was nothing I could do. I felt like my body had failed her. I wanted to hold her but I couldn't. She was on every drug known to humankind. She had IVs everywhere and she was on a ventilator. She had a chest bleed, brain bleeds, everything. She was on the extreme end of viability. By the third night, they said things weren't looking so good. She couldn't produce any urine. And I didn't want to act selfishly. Is she in pain? I wondered. I knew what it felt like as a grown woman with IVs and everything and it felt like hell. We had to make some rapid adjustments. We had dreams and plans for her. I had bought a Yale T-shirt from my alma mater, and Kevin had bought a hat from his, Brown University. But now all we wanted to do was to make this child as comfortable as possible. My dad gave me a music box and I put it on top of her Isolette. There's just so little you can do. We just wanted her to know that so many people were praying for her. They called and said that I should come down because she was going. When I got there I saw the numbers going down on the monitor. I asked them to turn them off. They started unhooking her and they wrapped her up and let me hold her. It was the first time I got to hold her. It was the first time I got to see her without all the tubes and stuff. She had a perfectly round head. She was still warm. I thought she looked like Kevin and she looked like she was smiling a little bit. Kevin got to hold her for a while; so did my mom and dad. It's one of those experiences you don't ever think will happen to you. We know it does happen, but we don't expect that it will happen to us. The experience of losing her was really intense. Your hopes are gone. Your plans for being a mother are gone. You go from an expectant mother to a person in mourning. The people in the hospitals are remarkably incapable of handling these things—which is sad when you realize that people die there all the time. I remember being rolled out of the hospital, not pregnant anymore; my child's body was in the morgue, but my life had changed. Everything about it had changed. My baby never left the hospital with me.

People figured that because of the circumstances surrounding Grace's death, Erica was not a real mother or parent. "Just because she only lived four days doesn't mean I am not a parent. It doesn't mean that I didn't have the hopes, dreams, and expectations that every other parent has. You have the full suite of thoughts and feelings that you have for a child. People who experience a loss still have the totality of experience of any other parent. People say stuff and they really don't think."

If you have suffered a pregnancy loss there are some things you should know.

* No matter what well-meaning nurses, family members, and friends say, you will not feel better in a couple of days, weeks, or maybe even months. Your hurt may continue for years. True healing only occurs after the slow and necessary progression through the different stages of grief and mourning.
* Consider a service or memorial that can give you closure. Countless women said having a funeral or memorial service made the loss real. "At our memorial service, I told people not to be afraid to say her name. She is a real person," says one mother. Erica and Kevin had baby Grace cremated and held a small memorial service. They keep the ashes on the mantelpiece of their home.
* Understand that grieving for a child is very different from grieving for the loss of a parent or grandparent. When you

grieve for an older person, you grieve for the past, but with a child you grieve for the future. Be open to understanding that some healing strategies that you or others used may not necessarily work for you. This type of loss is unique. It is also important to know that healing does not mean forgetting. You will never forget your precious baby, and successful grieving ensures that there is always a place in your heart for him or her.

✳ You do not have to carry this burden alone. No doubt, you have a number of loved ones who would love to be there for you but just don't know how. They are afraid of saying or doing the wrong thing. Tell them honestly what they can do to help. Do not say, for example, "I am fine," when you are not fine. By allowing others to share in your pain and help you out, you will be comforted and they will feel less helpless and awkward.

✳ Do not feel as if you cannot make choices for yourself at this time. It's true this is probably not the best time to make rash decisions about your job and moving out of state, but you can and should be involved with decisions related to the death of your baby. If there are decisions regarding naming the baby, seeing the baby, arranging a memorial or other service, or taking care of things you bought for the nursery, be involved in these choices. Well-meaning people may try to shield you from these things as if they are protecting you. Phyllis, from Chicago, says one of her main regrets over the death of their baby was that they did not have a memorial service for their son. "In retrospect I think that would have helped us heal better," she says (hear more from Phyllis on page 212). Counselors say participating in these decisions helps make the loss real. Until the loss is real, the grieving cannot begin. Instead of just painful thoughts, you can also have comforting memories of the kind and loving acts you did for your baby.

✳ It is probably true that you will be hurt, angry, or jealous if you are around mothers who have young babies. You may feel resentment and secretly wish ill on others. These are very real feelings for a person in the throes of grief. You are not a horrible person for thinking such thoughts. Be willing to forgive yourself, knowing that these feelings will eventually go away.

✳ Prepare yourself for a changed relationship with your spouse or partner. In some instances, these types of traumatic experiences can make two people closer. But sometimes there is resentment, anger, or blame secretly or openly brewing. If you sense this is happening to you, do not ignore it or assume it will get better with time. Find a grief counselor or a support group with other couples who have had a similar loss (see Appendix).

"We have to find a better way to look at a pregnancy that doesn't result in a bouncing baby boy or girl, so you don't feel like a failure. It is not a dark secret or shame. It becomes a failure that you speak of again. My friends had a memorial service for their daughter who died before birth, and they named her too. My friends said, don't be afraid to say her name; she is a real person," Erica says.

ReTell Therapy

MORE THAN THE BLUES

by Jeanne Whitfield

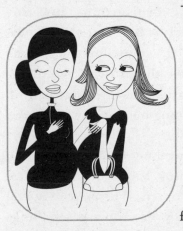

When I found out I was pregnant I was very depressed. This was not the plan; we were not supposed to have a third child. We had two children ages four and two, and I felt challenged caring for them. My plans did not include starting all over again with another baby. My feelings of depression over what should have been joyous news made me feel ashamed. I felt anything but joy.

On top of it all, the timing was terrible in many ways. Financially, it couldn't have been worse, we had already given away all of our baby things, and our home was not big enough to accommodate a third child. My husband was immediately aware of the fact that I was not happy about this. I was crying when I showed him the home pregnancy test, and they were not tears of joy. I kept telling him I would be fine, but I wasn't. I didn't want to leave the house; I would have emotional, sometimes angry outbursts. I wanted to stay in bed, even though I had two young children to care for, and that made me feel guilty as well. I feigned excitement when we told people and pretended to be happy when friends asked. I was ashamed of how I felt.

Finally, I broke down and told my husband just how upset I really was. I expected him to be disappointed in me or upset, but he wasn't; he was very kind and reassuring. He told me it was all right and that he knew it would be hard, but that I could do it. He told me he knew I had the ability to adapt and handle the responsibility of caring for a third child. His confidence in me was reassuring, but I was still upset about the situation. I prayed for peace of mind and strength to accept this change to our lives. I soon came to realize that I could do this; I had the strength and help I needed.

My advice is to talk to someone you trust—your mate, a close relative, or a trusted friend. Depression and desperation can cloud your ability to see a situation for what it really is. We are only able to see the negative that we are feeling; the positive gets lost somewhere along the way. Don't let your feelings of grief over this unexpected event overshadow the joy you can feel. The moment we took our newest little addition home, my feelings of depression and anxiety vanished. She was beautiful and precious and perfect, and how could I do anything but love and care for her. I did have enough love, ability, strength—everything I needed.

My husband is my hero. He saw in me what I couldn't see in myself. I hope that any woman who finds herself feeling the same way will not let feelings of shame allow her to hide behind false happiness or closed doors. You have to take hold of the negative feelings, not let them control you. Let the love that you have within, the love that created this little baby inside of you, the love that belongs to that precious baby, shine through.

ReTell Therapy

WEEPING FOR ADAM:
PREGNANCY AFTER A STILLBIRTH

by Phyllis Baldwin

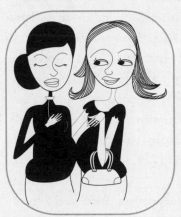

On December 30, 1997, I lay in a hospital bed with my husband and daughter by my side waiting for the birth and death of my son Adam. I was twenty-two weeks pregnant. My water broke about an hour after I arrived at the hospital and my obstetrician informed me that Adam would not live. His lungs were not mature enough for him to survive outside the womb. Prior to getting pregnant with Adam, my husband and I tried for eight years to conceive. This pregnancy meant so much to us. Now as I lay there waiting for the inevitable, I wondered why.

Why this was happening to us? What sins had we committed together or separately that we were being punished for? We were both healthy, well-educated, and financially secure. Both of us grew up in loving families and we were high school sweethearts. We were great parents to our eight-year-old daughter, Blair. So why wouldn't God bless us with another child? *We* loved children and had always planned on having a large family.

My obstetrician could not provide us with a reason for my late-term miscarriage. Her only advice was for us was to try again. I felt confused, sad, defeated, and empty. Try again? I couldn't. I thought maybe God was trying to tell me something; like maybe one kid is enough. Besides, I knew that getting pregnant again could not replace the loss of Adam. Lives are not interchangeable. My husband and I decided to put that part of our lives behind us.

Less than a year later, in August 1998, I was pregnant again. I was shocked and scared. I decided right away not to get emotionally involved in the pregnancy. I found a new obstetrician and began with my prenatal care. I didn't tell anyone that I was pregnant, except close friends and family, until I started to show. I wouldn't let myself think about the sex of the baby or names for the baby. My obstetrician suspected I might have a weak cervix and began to monitor it. Sure enough, my cervix began to dilate and I was rushed into outpatient surgery to have a cerclage, a surgical procedure to stitch the cervix closed. The news of my weak cervix, often called an incompetent cervix, answered my question as to why Adam died.

I still held in my emotions as my baby and belly grew. I was afraid of getting hurt again and I wasn't confident that the pregnancy would be a success. When I reached my seventh month, I began to relax because I knew if the baby was born now, he or she would have a good chance to survive. The day I delivered my healthy, full-term, eight-pound, four-ounce baby girl was bittersweet. I felt blessed and overwhelmed with grief. The entire pregnancy was overshadowed by Adam's death. Having a healthy baby after the death of another baby doesn't ease the feelings of loss, but it is a constant reminder of how fragile life is and how good God has been to me and my family.

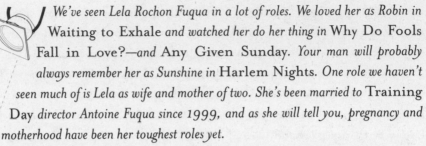

Spotlight On . . .
Lela Rochon, Little Boy Lost

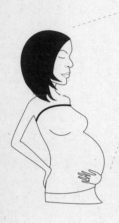

We've seen Lela Rochon Fuqua in a lot of roles. We loved her as Robin in Waiting to Exhale *and watched her do her thing in* Why Do Fools Fall in Love?—*and* Any Given Sunday. *Your man will probably always remember her as Sunshine in* Harlem Nights. *One role we haven't seen much of is Lela as wife and mother of two. She's been married to* Training Day *director Antoine Fuqua since 1999, and as she will tell you, pregnancy and motherhood have been her toughest roles yet.*

My pregnancy story does not begin as one of those happy-go-lucky stories. I just want to tell it honestly. Five months into my first pregnancy, my water broke while at work. It was 4:00 P.M. I had to deliver a little boy, but he was too young to survive. It never occurred to me that something so terrible would happen to me. I was healthy physically. I was athletic. But I was working too much and I was stressed. A week before I lost the baby, I was at the Golden Globes smiling and grinning on the red carpet. I didn't realize how stressed I was.

The point is that losing a child changes everything you feel and do from there. After that, the next pregnancy was pins and needles for me and everyone around me. Anytime relatives received a late night phone call, they worried I had bad news. But the second pregnancy was really a perfect pregnancy. I didn't have a day of morning sickness or any other real problems. Probably the biggest problem was me. You always feel that it is your fault when something happens. But I just tried to do everything I was told to do. At five months, they stitched my cervix closed, and told me to lie down flat or on my side but really never on my uterus, until it was over. It was hard, but I did it. I just lay there and waited on God, believing that he wouldn't be that cruel twice. And after I made it past twenty-eight weeks—when they say a baby can survive outside the womb—then I was okay. But I wasn't okay until then.

The most important thing women should realize is that you must listen to your body. I didn't listen to my body with the first pregnancy. The night before I lost the baby, I crawled up the stairs thinking that I wouldn't make it because I was so tired. I was working sixteen-hour days. I was extremely unhappy on the cable network show and they weren't respectful of my pregnancy. I couldn't even find my chair to sit down in between takes. I finally made it up the stairs that night, and I lay down. The next day I went to work and my water broke. You have to listen to your body.

As black women, it's not always easy for us to say, "No," or "I can't." But if I could give up the so-called success—the TV shows, the movies, or whatever—to have that baby back, I would do so in a second. So I was forced to say, I can't do this anymore. I basically gave up acting for motherhood, and it's a decision I have no regrets about. It's definitely hard to have a talent burning inside of you that you want to express and you can't because you're doing something else, but this is an incredible part of womanhood and life. To me, having children is just more important than anything. I understand it's not so for everybody, but it is for me.

That's why, for me, the best advice I got was to get back on the horse and try again. After the loss, I had surgery to have fibroids removed. The doctors don't know and will never know if the fibroids affected my miscarriage, but I had them removed. Six months later I got pregnant again. I know everybody's situation is different, but I also think you never truly get over that kind of loss and you never trust your body again until you see a healthy child come. When my daughter came and she was healthy and happy, it made everything okay.

And so after my daughter, Asia, I tried yet again. With my daughter I didn't have a day of morning sickness, but with my last pregnancy, my son, I was sick for about four and a half months. Plus, I was hungry every three hours around the clock. And I was so busy with this active toddler I didn't do all the things I did for myself before. With Asia, I totally pampered myself; I got massages twice a week at home, I had a manicurist and pedicurist come to my house—I was on bed rest at the time so it helped pass the day away.

You really need that so you don't go crazy on bed rest. I watched a lot of TV; I was on the computer a lot, and read a lot of books. I really got into nesting mode and decorated my whole nursery from my bed by telephone and Internet.

Now I tell every pregnant woman to get some sleep and get organized. Do everything you need to do so you can be rocking and waiting in that chair. Be ready, because your life will never be the same.

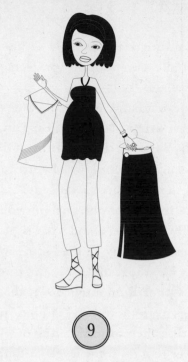

9

Mocha Style

How to Look Like a Babe
When You're Having One

Pregnancy clothes have come a long way. We've gone from garish collars and muumuus to belly-bearing tops and racy maternity lingerie. The biggest problem used to be finding something that wasn't ghastly to wear; now your biggest problem is sifting through all the high-end and low-end Internet sites and specialty stores. Or should you just buy one of those mix-and-match collections with an entire maternity wardrobe in one box? Do you like your maternity pants to fit above the belly or below the belly? These days we're spoiled for choice, and we're paying dearly for it given the eye-popping price tags on some of the maternity gear.

But that still doesn't help me figure out what to wear. The choices seem endless: Mimi Maternity, Liz Lange, Pea in the Pod, Japanese Weekend, Barney's Procreation, Old Navy, the Gap, Motherhood Maternity, Pumpkin Maternity, and Duo from JCPenney. Phew! I'm out of breath and there's more to the list. A pregnant woman definitely has options, but you still have to figure out what you actually really need and what is just the extra stuff.

When it comes to maternity clothes some women can't wait to get into them. They buy the jeans, tops, and underwear before they are even showing. Other women go down that road kicking and screaming, hanging on to their usual clothes until every fiber and thread are stretched to the point of crying out for mercy.

I'm a firm believer that on some level—and please don't get deep and philosophical on me here—it is the clothes that make the woman. By that I mean, when you look good, you feel good. Enter pregnancy.

Even the most card-carrying fashionista—you know, the one who looks well put together every day—can find pregnancy a little challenging. One obstacle is time, or the lack thereof. You may not have the extra time in the morning to contemplate deeply which of your forty-five pairs of shoes best brings out the subtle crimson hues in your blouse.

What you need, my dear, is a pregnancy style. Everyone has a style—even if it's athletic, casual, or preppy. Most of us don't give much thought to categorizing our style; we just get dressed every day. Even if you don't think you have one, you do. Black women are known purveyors of exceptional style. And although the white history books want us to believe that our African ancestors were uncivilized savages, we absolutely know better. The fourteenth- and fifteenth-century African empires of Ghana, Mali, Egypt, Kush, and others developed fabrics and jewelry from indigenous resources. Other tribes used skins of leather from leopards and goats to make clothing. A report from a historic pilgrimage by a Malian king states that many of the twelve thousand servants, slaves, and companions with him donned clothing made of silk and brocade. And though the invading white missionaries convinced the world that the Africans' tendency to wear minimal clothing was another sign of their savagery, we know (because it's painfully obvious) that the clothes were suited for the hot climates.

Just as our ancestors did, black women, through the years, have created their own grassroots style based on their needs, feelings, and communities instead of following what fashion designers dictate. One study showed that almost a third of all black women are fashion innovators, compared to less than one-sixth of all other women. In the same survey, 57 percent of black women said they would prefer to be slightly overdressed than underdressed for a party, compared to 44 percent of all other women. Given the impressive percentage of fashion-conscious sisters, it is no wonder that that grungy, disheveled, just-jumped-out-of-bed look has never been accepted among any of the descendents of the diaspora.

Instead, we remember our mamas getting dressed up for church in their Sunday best and church hats. We were raised with an appreciation for being neat and clean. And if you're like me, you probably got more than one spanking for messing up your Sunday shoes or playing in your "school" clothes and not your "play" clothes. Plus, we grew up with the added pressure of being tidy and fresh so white folks wouldn't know we were poor. Many times my mother stopped me at the door with a "I know you don't think you're going out the house like *that*!" This was especially true after all those years in predominantly white schools made me think it was okay to go to school with dirty jeans, a T-shirt, and some sneakers. But my mother was not having it. And it was my mother, with her old-fashioned values (she still can't accept that I don't wear pantyhose) and her classic style, who taught me the value of a scarf, a special brooch, and, most importantly, walking with my head held up high—the most stylish fashion accessory of them all.

Diahann Carroll, our sophisticated icon, was the first black woman to have a signature clothing line, in 1997. We've come a long way, fashionably speaking, since then, with lines from Eve, Beyoncé, and the phenomenal empire of BabyPhat under the stewardship of Kimora Lee Simmons (hear Kimora's take on pregnancy style on page 237). Our men have broken barriers as well with FUBU, Sean John, Phat Farm, and others—in fact, it seems that every black Tom, Dick, and Harry of the music and entertainment world is launching a clothing line.

Meanwhile, Halle Berry, Beyoncé, Mary J. Blige, Missy Elliott, Alicia Keys, and Patti LaBelle continue our iconic style legacy, picking up where Dorothy Dandridge, Lena Horne, Ella Fitzgerald, and others left off.

So, girl, you are oozing in a stylish past and present that is rich and deep. Try to remember this when you feel you'll only look good in a circus tent, and you're staring at a mound of clothes that you've ripped off in disgust as you can't find one single item of clothing that you don't feel ridiculous in.

But how do you tap into your stylish pregnancy self? Take heart, my love; your style is probably right under your nose. Or under those bodacious boobs you're carrying around. Whatever you do, pregnancy is not the time to reinvent yourself drastically. With all the crazy things going on with your body and your life, you need to feel that *you're still you*, at least on some levels. If you can't figure out your style, think of someone whose look is similar to yours and go from there.

There's traditional—think Brooks Brothers and Talbots—classic, artsy, trendy, or easygoing casual. If that doesn't help, think store style. Now that my shopping time is limited, I'm a Banana Republic kind of girl, with a little Bebe and a few designer splurges, like Tracey Reese and Escada, thrown in. I have friends who love the look of Express and can walk in and get their entire wardrobe for the season. And if you're still at a loss, ask a girlfriend. Or even a guy. I am a diehard for three things—high-heeled shoes and boots, a pair of tailored black trousers, and form-hugging boot-cut jeans. My pregnancy wardrobe has always maintained these basics. My other passions are handbags and jewelry, and you'll quickly learn the importance of accessories when you're pregnant. But more on that later; right now, we have to get you to identify your style.

As we take this style journey, my premise is simple. First, you should not compromise your style just because you're pregnant unless your style is one that needs to be eighty-sixed anyway. Second, clothes should show off, not hide your body. I'm not saying you have to show your belly to the world (though if you're comfortable, go with it!), but fitted clothes make you look thinner and send a message to the world that pregnancy is beautiful, natural, and downright sexy! Last, you don't need Kimora Lee Simmons's budget to have a wonderful wardrobe. We'll focus on a few key pieces, with a few optional splurges along the way that can get you through work, weekends, evening, travel, holidays, and special occasions.

The first thing you should do is take a personal inventory. Go closet shopping to find how many of your own things can still be worn during pregnancy. Your inventory should include:

1. Blazers. Do not wear your man's jacket, under any circumstances (there are other items in his closet we will raid). The proportions are all wrong and will make you look like a linebacker for the Dallas Cowboys.
2. Button-down shirts/blouses.
3. Sweaters.
4. T-shirts.
5. Ribbed turtlenecks and other knit shirts.
6. Stretchy pants (any Lycra blend).
7. Drawstring or elastic waistband pants.
8. Wrap dresses/skirts.
9. Solid color dresses with simple lines.

The more pieces you find from your closet inventory, the less you'll have to buy. You can also borrow maternity clothes from friends and relatives. Nanette, an office manager in the Dayton, Ohio, area, and her friends keep a rotating collection of maternity clothes. When someone in the sister circle is done with her maternity clothes, any gently used items go into a box that stays at Nanette's house. You can start your own maternity collection system and use it to help stretch any maternity pieces you do buy. Now that you know what you have and what you don't, it's time to go shopping. Right? Wrong!

THE FIRST TRIMESTER

If this is your first baby, you'll probably skate through your first trimester without a visit to the maternity store, unless you're just dying to go. OK, OK, I have to admit, I loved going to the maternity stores when I didn't really need them, for a chance to play around with those fake tummies they have in the dressing room, just to get an idea of what I would look like a few months down the road. It takes about twelve weeks for the uterus to rise out of the pelvis, so even if you feel bloated and are peeing all the time, the only thing that is oversized right now are your boobs. Wearing a maternity shirt at this point will only make you look bigger. And since you don't know how big you'll actually get, buying maternity clothes in the early days can be a waste of money. You may want to pick up a few things in the regular store but about two sizes bigger. Make a few reconnaissance trips to the maternity shops, but with a few tricks you can probably skip actually buying anything at the maternity store.

Trick 1: Extend the life of your favorite jeans or pants. When you're at the stage when you feel a little bloated, or worse, you leave the house feeling comfortable but by the time lunch is done, your pants are so tight you can't wait to get back to your desk and open the button and zipper, try carrying a ponytail elastic in your bag at all times. You can easily make a dash to the bathroom, loop the elastic around the button, pull the rest of it through your button-hole, and pull it back over to loop around the button again.

When things get really bad you can swap the ponytail holder for a large rubber band—the kind you get from an office supply store or off your Sunday newspaper. Thread it through the buttonhole and wrap it around the button. It can make your favorite pants last a lot longer. Just don't let the rubber band touch your skin. Wear a T-shirt tucked in, and a large shirt over it to cover your little secret.

The Second Trimester

The beginning of the second trimester is still a little tricky, because you may be too small for full-blown maternity clothes and too big for all your usual clothes. Your mocha girlfriends will tell you to ramp it up to the bigger stuff and be comfortable. You may still be able to get away with larger sizes of "normal" clothes. Depending on your husband's size you can borrow a few button-down shirts to pair with some jeans or black trousers. I remember looking at my husband's shirt thinking how big it was, and two blinks later it was too small. By the end of it all, I couldn't button the shirt all the way to the bottom and my husband was complaining that I was ruining all his shirts. I promptly showed him the $168 price tag on the black blazer I bought from Liz Lange, and he quickly shut up and offered me more shirts. This works with most men.

But most of us need full-blown maternity clothes by the second trimester. Before you whip out the debit card, do a little exploration and price comparisons, and don't forget reasonably priced chains like Wal-Mart, Target, and Old Navy, which can carry items similar to the pricey boutiques. Also check out some of the plus-size stores; plus-size clothing is really stylish these days and the stores are great places to find elastic band pants and roomy, longer tops.

Before you buy, think about your lifestyle. Do you work in a professional environment where you need a suit or something close to it every day? Do you stay at home? What about your weekends? Entertaining? Church? Hitting the hot spots with your girlfriends? Are there any weddings or cocktail parties in the upcoming months? Here are some general tips:

1. When starting out, go to a smaller boutique rather than a large department store. The salespeople at smaller boutiques can provide more hands-on assistance, offer suggestions, and help get you properly measured for a bra. They tend to have great ideas and stories from other moms-to-be about tips to expand a wardrobe.
2. Buy a little bit at a time. Start with basics like black pants, jeans, khakis, and leggings, along with sweaters or T-shirts, depending on the season, in neutral colors that are versatile.
3. Try to get maternity versions of what you have in your closet now.
4. Think mix-and-match tops, pants, blazers, and sweaters to maximize your wardrobe.

Work

Dressing for the job is always pregnancy challenge number one. It's hard to command respect and work your best power presentation when you're worried that your clothes don't fit. It's so easy to look sloppy when you're pregnant that you have to put more thought into looking well-put-together and polished. If you have a high-profile job, or work in an office with a stated or unstated dress code, you may need to invest in some high-quality office wear pieces.

All the sister CEOs, or sister CEOs in training, or those who just have the kind of job that requires you to wear a suit every day, may have to bite the bullet here and buy a maternity suit. If you buy the dress, the pants and/or skirt, and the jacket, you'll have a number of options to work with. Remember, you're the only one in the world who expects a pregnant woman to wear something new every day. The trick is to wear the same suit, but alter the blouse or accessories to give it a fresh look. The jacket is always the most important part of the suit, so go for soft tailoring. You can't lose with a simple single-breasted suit. The look is slimming (take all the help you can get!) and helps reduce the appearance of wider hips and big breasts. Charcoal gray is the most versatile color. Just got your tax refund or won a scratch-off lottery? Splurge for a long dress coat to top the look. Pair it with a knee-length dress or skirt, and you can't lose.

Trick 1: To avoid blowing a wad of money on suits you'll never wear again, there are a number of places on the Internet that rent out maternity "careerwear"—pantsuits and dresses and special occasion dresses. Nicole, a pharmaceutical sales rep from Los Angeles, spent about one hundred dollars a month for up to five outfits and had a fresh look every thirty days. Denise from Manassus, Virginia, also went the leasing route and loved it. She says the moral boost of looking hot and "on point" at work was worth the investment. At most of these sites, you receive a discount on future leases and any renewals.

Trick 2: If you can't find anything that fits as well as your favorite black pants, create your own homemade maternity panel. Buy one from a fabric or notions store for a couple of dollars and take it to a seamstress to have it sewn in (the instructions are usually on the package). If you can, get busy with a sewing machine and do it yourself. But remember that once the maternity panel goes in, you can't get those pants back. My petite friend Shanice, who always has trouble finding the perfect fit, did this with her favorite Express trousers, knowing she could always go back to the store postpregnancy and get some more.

Here are some tips for other pieces:

Fitted jackets: You can probably still wear some of your favorite jackets, unbuttoned, of course, for most of this trimester. A jacket over a fitted top works really well. A nice black jacket can make almost any outfit look like it means business.

Pants: Leave the palazzo pants alone. Go for cigarette pants, which are slim, with a slight boot cut for a great look.

Dresses: If you wear dresses, then you must have a wrap dress. It's a classic style created by Diane von Furstenberg, and it's surprisingly versatile, fluid, and perfect for pregnant bodies. I had a black wrap dress that I wore to death. I wore it to work, with a neat scarf tied at my neck. Add some funky jewelry to jazz it up, or add chandelier earrings (hair pulled back), a pashmina shawl, and some really cute shoes for an evening look. Another basic is a straight sleeveless knit shift dress in black or gray. This can also be paired with a jacket for work and worn with a chunky choker in the evening.

A major caveat about dresses: if you go the nonmaternity dress route, remember that as your belly gets bigger, the front of the dress gets shorter than the back. This is not a cute look. And unless the dress reaches down to the ankles, you will indeed have this effect. The only suggestion besides stop stonewalling and go to the maternity store is to have a tailor lengthen the front about a quarter inch, while leaving the back untouched.

Sweaters: Sweaters are a must-have when pregnant, office girl or not. First of all, you always need to have one handy for when your hormone-induced hot flash just as quickly turns into a freezing moment. A button-down cardigan with a V neck and an "open" bottom that hangs is a great help at the office on those casual Fridays. It's also a great piece and can be substituted for a blazer, paired with a lacy camisole, loose oxford shirt, or basic tee. Go for deep solid colors like black, navy, or charcoal gray. These are more versatile with your wardrobe and more—our favorite word— slimming than brighter colors.

Pantyhose: Don't assume you have to buy the maternity kind just yet. Try the less expensive queen size version for your height. But definitely do something. There's nothing worse than trying to work at your desk as your stockings are cutting off your circulation.

Layering: Layering is a most important word for pregnancy style. When you're pregnant, you are almost always hot—even if you're sitting buck naked on a large pack of peas in the frozen food aisle. I was pregnant throughout the winter and I was always sweating— even in strange places like under my breasts. What I now know, and wish I knew through my two pregnancies, is that layering is the antidote. Style experts and sweat reduction gurus agree that you should start with a T-shirt, then add a blouse or shirt, and on top of that a sweater. You can always tie the sweater around your neck. Even in the summertime, it's nice to have something to throw on when you get one of those arctic blasts from the mall and some restaurants.

Casual wear: This is where we have a lot of fashion casualties. See, the thing about work clothes is that although they are more expensive to maintain, it's a uniform: pants, top, jacket; skirt, top, jacket; dress and jacket; et cetera, et cetera. But when you don't have the structure of a uniform, you can sort of lose it. Remember when casual Fridays started and you would see all of those cartoons about people who took it to extremes? Better yet, those coworkers at your job who confused Casual Fridays with Dirty Clothes Fridays, or No-Need-to-Iron Fridays; well, it's kind of like that. When going casual, try to maintain a together look. You don't have to resort to sweat pants and big T-shirts. And, please, don't leave your house with leggings and your husband's button-down shirt thing. It's a passé look that makes you appear larger on top and it's like a major fashion don't.

Instead, stick with two casual basics: a good pair of jeans and some comfortable black trousers, like a pair of loose-fitting yoga pants (sisters swear by these!). Yoga pants can easily convert from pajamas to loungewear. Jeans can be dressed up or down. Add a sexy tank or a fitted tee with a V neckline (show that cleavage, girl!) and some cute heels for a casual night out to dinner and a movie with your husband or girlfriends. Add a button-down shirt for running errands or other weekend activities.

PREGNANCY AND SUMMERTIME:
A DREADED COMBINATION

If you are pregnant and in a locale with hot summers, I feel for you, girl. I was born in August, and give my mother a lot of respect for being nine months in the hottest month of the year in New York City. Summer is such a problem because most pregnant women are already having their own personal summer anyway. Plus, you have the typical worries of dehydration, heat stroke, and exhaustion. Here are some tips:

1. Wear light fabrics that breathe and don't cling to your body.
2. If your arms are still jiggling five seconds after you stopped moving them, you may want to consider short sleeves instead of sleeveless. If you must go sleeveless, try wide-neck tanks, which draw attention to your neck and face. If those are bloated beyond recognition, too, then I suggest staying indoors. Just kidding.
3. T-shirts with those three-quarter sleeves that almost get to the elbows are also a possibility.

Even though the heat is a challenge, summer is one of the easiest seasons for pregnancy dress. The only dreaded summer dilemma is whether to wear shorts or not to wear shorts. Both times I was pregnant, my thighs did a lot of growing. I mean really growing. Forget thunder thighs; I had the thunder-lightning-and-category-four-hurricane-thighs. I was sure I could have sparked a forest fire with the friction I created from walking. In this case, it is very difficult to find flattering shorts. With my ample thighs and my big butt, all of my maternity shorts turned into a mangled mess in between my legs—not a good look. So if you have been spared the thigh spreadage, go right ahead with the shorts. Take this simple test: Put on a pair of pantyhose and take a walk. If you can hear the sound of your thighs rubbing together, you probably shouldn't wear shorts. If you can wear shorts, wear short shorts: not the Daisy

Duke sort that look like you've been shopping in Lil' Kim's closet, but something midthigh. Since the rest of my legs still looked great, I found a cute denim mini skirt that lasted all summer. Pair it with a halter top (great support too!) or any sort of tank top, and you can't lose.

Capri pants are a pregnant woman's best friend in the spring and summer months, and some of fall too. It's hard to go wrong with a pair of capris and a tee, sleeveless shirt, V-neck top, or light sweater. Capris can be supercasual with some flat thong sandals or kicked up a notch with a low-heel mules.

Evening/Special Occasion

There's nothing more frustrating than a close friend who is so self-ish, she decides to get married while you're pregnant. Here's my cardinal rule about friendship: friends don't get married when their other friends are thirty to forty pounds overweight and can't do anything about it. My girlfriend Schalawn got married when I was about seven months pregnant with my second child, and I looked about the way a first-time preggie looks at nine months of pregnancy. I'm still working out my forgiveness issues with Schalawn, as my pudgy face and teetering waddle are now forever immortalized in her wedding album and video. I have other regrets about my appearance at Schalawn's wedding, too; I could have done much better with my outfit. Here's what I wish I would have remembered: whenever you have a dressup emergency or last-minute formal, cocktail party, or black tie affair to attend, you can never go wrong with a simple, slinky black dress, and a dressy shawl or wrap. The dress should be soft with fluid lines, and your wrap can be shimmery, or a contrasting color that says WOW! Add some to-die-for strappy shoes and a cute purse and you are good to go!

You can also rent a special occasion dress from one of the Internet sites or turn a work pantsuit into a sophisticated statement by adding a nice lacy camisole, some killer jewelry, a stylish evening bag, and some open-toe shoes (pedicure required).

If you plan on buying one dressy piece, make sure it's black.

That saying Black is beautiful doesn't just apply to you. It applies to all pregnant women because black is slimming, and when you're pregnant, my friends, slimming is about as beautiful as you can get.

Another surprising option is a tube top—a maternity tube top, that is. It's longer to cover the tummy fully. I saw a sister working one at a banquet I attended. It was black (of course!) and paired with some dressy black pants and some nice silver jewelry. The outfit was so nice I didn't even check to see the flab factor on her arms.

If you've got style chutzpah, off-the-shoulder necklines also work well. They are said to accentuate and lengthen the neck while playing up your décolletage without making you look like Pamela Anderson. Here are some more must-haves:

Accessories

* Wraps and shawls are a pregnant woman's best friend. The dressier the occasion, the longer the shawl, if you ask me. And when it's time for a black tie affair or ball, a floor-length wrap is absolutely spectacular. An oblong scarf can be tossed over your shoulder for a nice evening look that is romantic and feminine. Wrap it around your neck a few times and let it go!
* Scarves. A pocket square scarf folded long and straight and then loosely tied around the neck is a great way to add color around your face without doing the big scarf thing.
* Inexpensive, fun jewelry.
* Bangles.
* Sunglasses: Think Hollywood glamour.
* Handbags: If it's just for everyday schlepping around, think of something that's comfortable on your shoulders, arms, and back. Our bags are typically brimming with all sorts of things anyway, and now that you're pregnant, you've likely tossed in some snacks, a bottle of water, and a pregnancy book (this one, I hope!) to read. That can make a bag really heavy. Be careful: an overloaded bag can damage your back and your posture. If you're having back problems, consider a backpack. There are a

number of cute ones, and you'll get some use out of it later when your baby arrives, since backpacks, and the freed hands they create, are a must when dealing with little ones.

Shoes

There's a big myth circulating the streets that pregnant women should wear flats. My husband used to drive me nuts with his constant reminders that I should be wearing flats. Actually a thick, chunky heel gives you the structure and support you need during your pregnancy. Any doctor worth his prenatal vitamins will tell you wearing sneakers every day is not necessarily the best move for pregnant women. It seems like everytime I saw my mother, she would look at my heels and say, "Are you sure you're supposed to be wearing *those*?" My response was always the same: "Absopositutely." Kimora Lee Simmons was another shoe diehard, unwilling to let her stilettos go until the bitter end. Of course, with all her money, chauffeurs, and curbside treatment, I'm sure she wasn't actually walking very much in those numbers. Stilettos may be a no-no, but you don't have to abandon heels altogether as long as you're comfortable.

Since feet have been known to grow during pregnancy, you may have to buy a new pair of shoes during these nine months. Do yourself a favor: find something you will actually wear after pregnancy since there is a high probability that your foot will not return to its prepregnancy size. I'm sorry, but you bought this book to hear the truth.

The Third Trimester: Fashion in the Final Stretch

Trick 1: If you get to the point that your shirts and blouses don't cover your stomach anymore or if you're just itching for a different look under a blazer or cardigan, try this idea I stole from my mom. Make a scarf shirt. Mommy calls hers a dickie, but I think you have to be over fifty-five to use that word. Take a medium-sized silk scarf, iron it nicely, and sew on a piece of elastic from the top left corner to the top right corner. Do this again on the bottom right corners, making sure you have enough elastic to reach over your belly. Voilà! you have a fresh shirt to wear. If you're in a pinch, you can actually safety pin the scarf to your bra (my mom does this all the time, under a suit). Pin it just above your cups, where the straps begin, and on the sides of the bra, below the cups. The pin-pinch-fix works better with a jacket that you can still close the top button, or else it could lead to an embarrassing moment.

Try as you might to maintain a celebrity style throughout your own pregnancy, there will be a time—and the celebrities in this book will tell you—when your desire to be comfortable trumps your desire to be cute. This usually happens at the end of the eighth month and beyond. During my second pregnancy, I impressed myself with my style. People stopped me on the street to compliment my style, and my girlfriends said I set a new standard for pregnancy cuteness. Men were even telling my husband how sexy I looked. But when I got to my ninth month, none of that stuff meant a hill of beans. My stomach was so big and freakishly pointy that even the extra-large tees at the maternity store couldn't fit over my stomach and cover the maternity panel of my jeans.

From about my seventh month, my fabulous mother sensed that I was bigger than my small frame could handle. For weeks, everytime I visited my parents, my mom offered me this ghastly red print 1950s housedress/muumuu type of garment that basically looked like a circus tent with short sleeves. I told her I would never be caught dead in something like that. Hello? I was a pregnancy fashionista to the end. (Hadn't she been an eyewitness to my hot outfits?) After weeks of prodding, I finally just put the darn thing in my bag. Girls, about two weeks before my delivery date, I was so huge and so uncomfortable that in an act of desperation I dug out the muumuu and put it on. It was frighteningly liberating and delightful. I never took it off until it was time to go to the hospital. Sure, I washed it. Once. And I stood there butt-naked leaning on the dryer waiting for it to finish. I had done my part to promote the stylish pregnancy thing and prove that pregnancy doesn't have to be a fashion horror story, but it was time to surrender. My gig was up.

To all you fellow fashionistas out there, there may be a time when you become unbearably big and uncomfortable. All of us understand if you want to dig out a tent, an oversized sweatshirt, or your husband's basketball jerseys, and just be comfortable. Go for it, with no regrets or bad feelings. Your mocha girls understand. In fact, the ones who chose comfort over fashion from the very beginning are probably having a good laugh right now, because when you get down to the final days of pregnancy-being a comfortista is a classic move that never goes out of style.

The IT List
The Top Ten Things No Pregnancy Wardrobe Should Be Without

1. Black pants.
2. Jeans.
3. Cardigan wrap sweater.
4. Maternity bra: Get professionally measured. It may be awkward to have a salesperson feel you up, but getting the right size makes you happier in the long run. The women who work in maternity boutiques or in the lingerie section of major department stores are very knowledgeable in this field.

* Once you find your size and style, give it a test run for a few days before stocking up.

* When you're sure it's a keeper, stock up. Buy at least three or four.

* If you have a tried-and-true supportive bra from, say, Victoria's Secret, there's no reason you can't get that same bra in a bigger cup size.

* If you were stacked before you got pregnant, you should go to a maternity store, where they usually have large-size bras.

5. Comfortable hosiery and underwear—thong, G-strings, or the granddaddy of them all, the oversized over-the-belly panties: whatever is comfortable works.

6. Fitted T-shirts.

7. Wrap dress.

8. A crisp white button-down shirt—always looks good with black trousers, denim jeans, or a slim skirt. Feeling funky? Undo the last few buttons and tie it up over your belly.

9. Funky accessories to give a recycled outfit a fresh look.

10. A little black dress.

Dress Success
Style Tips to Flatter Every Girl's Body Type

We tend to come in thicker packages, and that's the way our men like us, thankyouverymuch. If you already have ample butt and hips, maternity clothes can be a real challenge. The designer says a particular size will last you for nine months, but right off the bat, your butt is taking up more space than those manufacturers ever planned for. As your tummy grows, your butt obviously gets jealous and wants to get in on the fun. Hips spread a wee bit wider to make room for the cargo that's coming through in a few months. Sisters with more curves, or more junk in the trunk, should shop carefully to avoid wasting money on things that won't fit in six weeks. Try these general rules and some specifics for curvaceous mamas.

✳ Never trust those maternity sizing charts that base your maternity size on your prepregnancy size. Try on everything and assume nothing.

✳ Before you invest in an item, give it a pull to test the stretchiness of the fabric. If there isn't much extra pull, the item may not last the whole pregnancy.

Wider Hips

Avoid stretchy styles that hug all the wrong places. Try skirts and dresses with a hip-hiding A-line shape that is close at the waist and then slightly flares out. Or wear a halter, V-neck, or jewelry to draw attention up to your shoulders and chest and away from your midsection. Go for boot cut or slightly flared pants; they help balance out the look of wider hips. Wide necklines can balance wider hips.

Big butt

Minimize a generous bottom with wide-leg pants without any back pockets or detail that attracts attention to that area. Wear darker colors on the bottom or small prints to deemphasize your bottom. Wearing low-riding, hipsters, or under-the-belly low riders instantly makes your butt look smaller and accentuates your waistline. Avoid clingy fabrics, opting for lighter, sheer fabrics floating around your body to create an illusion of lightness.

Thicker Thighs: Wear color on top, a red shell, for example, to draw attention away from your legs. Go with A-line skirts. Flat-front pants will give you more room. If you have a favorite brand of trousers that works for you, have a maternity panel sewn in. Avoid tapered legs or any pant that reveals a size difference between the upper and lower leg. Choose jackets that are fitted or flare just above the thighs.

Fuller Figure: Resist the urge to hide under shapeless tentlike shirts and dresses. Look for a sexier style dress with draping to slim your silhouette. Try shirts that are a little longer. When a shirt sits lower at the hips, instead of around the waist, it gives a slender appearance. Stay away from large prints: the larger the print, the larger you look. Don't cut your outfit at the waist. Go for longer jackets, longer tops, and tunics that give a more slender appearance. Dress all in one color to give yourself a long, lean look.

Petite Frame: Avoid the straight, no-waist look. Go for a fitted dress and heels. Elongate your look with slim, cropped pants like capris or cigarette pants. Wear cuffless and flat-front pants since cuffs and pleats shorten the leg.

Mocha Mix: What the Sisters Say . . . About Pregnancy Style

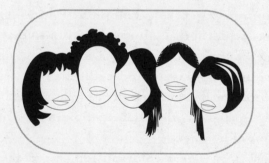

I tried to stick with my own style. I wore a lot of trousers and pant suits. I rented suits online for four weeks for about fifty bucks each. Then I would send those back and rent some more. I got about five suits every month and my look was always refreshed. I even rented some formal dresses for the Christmas parties. —Denise, Manassus, Virginia

I tried to really look good. I wore a lot of black and added color with my accessories—a really bold necklace or a scarf, shawl, or poncho. —Elizabeth, Jackson, Mississippi

I thought the Liz Lange collection at Target was really good. I would mix that up with some more expensive staples from the larger boutiques, and I was set. —ROCHELLE, STERLING, VIRGINIA

When you look at the expensive maternity clothes, maybe a cheap and cheerful muumuu isn't so bad after all. —DIANE, FREEPORT, NEW YORK

I did a lot with beautiful necklaces and earrings. I hoped it would draw attention up and away from my stomach. —DAVIA, CHERRY HILL, NEW JERSEY

SPOTLIGHT ON . . . KIMORA LEE SIMMONS, YOU BETTER WORK IT, GIRL!

"Who would want to have sex with a beast like me?" screamed Kimora Lee Simmons around the eighth month of her second pregnancy. Even former supermodels have a bad day. The creative director of Baby Phat and wife of hip-hop impresario Russell Simmons, Kimora is known as the Queen of Conspicuous Consumption with her extralong platinum Bentley and diamond flecked watches. But even she couldn't buy her way out of morning sickness or stretch marks. Kimora talks candidly about those pregnancy maladies, accepting her new body, being a pregnant diva, and the therapeutic benefits of a good cry.

When I became pregnant, I was so excited. I was newly married and wanted everything to be perfect. My goal was to cut out all the bull—and create a special, peaceful, stress-free space for my baby and me. Of course, this is easier said than done. For some reason, people always bring their drama to me. To cope, I flipped the diva switch, by screaming, "Oh my baby, you're stressing out my baby!" People respond to the baby's needs more than mine.

A lot of my pregnancy expectations were blown to bits. I dreamed of being vibrant, beautiful, and glowing all the time; instead I was extremely ill with morning sickness for the first three months. Even water made me sick. I ended up in the hospital because I was dehydrated. Because I am just a person of excess, I never tried a traditional suggestion like eat a small meal or eat crackers. First of all, I don't do crackers. I am not a parrot. And when I felt I could eat, I ate a big steak with all the fixin's. And then I got the paper bag for my head. Also, crazy things were going on with my body—a funny hair grew out of my boob, I was extremely clumsy, and I was often constipated. I even got stretch marks on my thighs. And, honey, don't waste your money on laser removal—it does not work. It just burns like hell and those suckers are still there.

At work I was under a lot of pressure to meet numbers. At times I felt like I couldn't go on. I was so stressed and overwhelmed I would just break down and cry. And cry some more. This was odd because I've always been a tough girl and not really a crier. But now I'm convinced there are definite medical and psychological benefits to crying. It was like a load was lifted and I could go on one more day.

When out, I exuded confidence and self-esteem. I would say, I'm beautiful and that giving life is so beautiful, and that is all very true. But I was also as big as three of me—prepregnancy. In my last trimester, I stopped doing any public events. I hated to see myself photographed. My expanding body was such a dramatic change for me. I've been modeling since age thirteen and have always been thin, a size zero. Being in the modeling industry, there's a way of thinking and a competitiveness about being thin that's ingrained in you and I wasn't immune to that. So that was a really big deal for me. I'm still struggling with my new body size and I've learned to accept that I may never be the old Kimora again.

My style has always been sexy, feminine, fresh, and classy. So when I was pregnant, I was not running around in Russell's sweatshirts. I was still me. I had great boobs and I fell in love with them. They were big as hell, and soft and hot in a way no boob job could ever give you, honey. My wardrobe basically accentuated my boobs and showed off my tummy. And I had to have my four-inch stilettos—girls, I just couldn't let those go.

There are two types of maternity girls—you're either an under the belly girl or a way over the belly girl. I was definitely, a strictly under the belly girl. Don't ever try to be an in the middle girl. It rarely looks right, and you're probably knocking your poor baby in the head with some elastic band. My goal was to be cute and comfortable—except for the shoes, of course. I wore a lot of slip dresses and anything stretchy and elastic from leggings to tank tops. Most of what I wore was custom-made by Baby Phat, and I would make some of my own stuff. I never really crossed over into legitimate maternity clothes; I would just buy larger sizes of, say, comfortable velours, and roll that waistband down under my belly. My only two maternity items were a pair of black trousers and a white button-down shirt that my girlfriend got for me. They were both great.

As you know, I'm a shopaholic. And the whole hormonal imbalance thing just sent me over the edge. At the end of both pregnancies, I probably had more than fifty pairs of jeans and about seventy-five blouses. I know it was wrong. But since they were regular clothes in large sizes I rationalized that I could take them all in and continue wearing them postpregnancy. That never happened.

And then there were the jewelry binges. My fingers and wrists expanded and I kept buying bigger watches, rings, and bracelets. I told myself they would be future gifts for my children, but it was all unnecessary and hormone-induced.

I definitely recommend a matte jersey black dress as a wardrobe staple. In the winter I wore stretchy turtlenecks, and I always had a good cashmere coat. My best pregnancy style advice is to work it, girl! Stick with what you know and a style that you usually wear. Honey, pregnancy is no time to tread into uncharted territory.

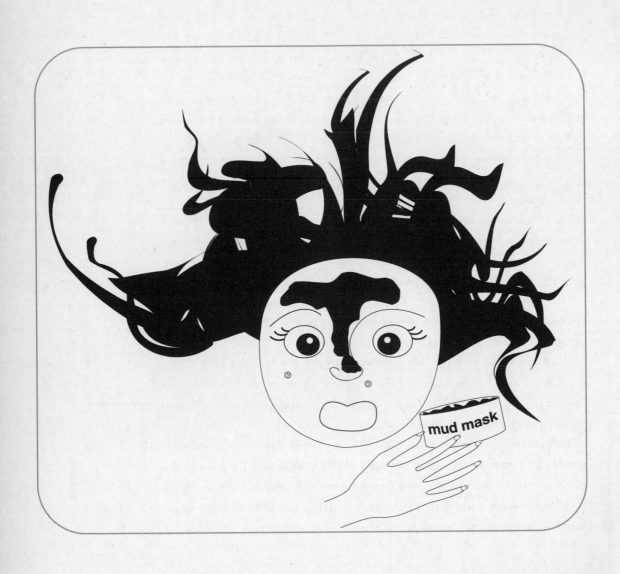

10

The Mocha Fix

SOLUTIONS FOR YOUR HAIR, SKIN, AND
NAIL PROBLEMS

Nothing can wreck the flow of your fabulous pregnancy more than hair, skin, and nail issues. After all, we are black women, and, historically, looking good is very important to us. Didn't Madame C. J. Walker, the first black female self-made millionaire in the United States, reach that standing by selling makeup and hair care products?

Now, let's be clear—you are always beautiful in pregnancy. After all, you are carrying around a life, and that's the ultimate fashion accessory.

Unfortunately, we live in a society in which the standard of beauty is still European. We've come a long way, but we ain't there yet. And I also know that a lot of our sisters still struggle to feel attractive and valued. The way we look plays into our self-esteem. Sadly, some women are even pushed to a level of obsession over their hair, skin tone, and body size and shape. Studies show that dissatisfaction with one's own natural beauty can lead to a lack of confidence in relationships, your work life, and yourself. Researchers have found that black women who internalize mainstream beauty ideals are more likely to be depressed than those who do not. Instead of being depressed about the person you are not, celebrate the person you are. Black women are oozing with natural beauty: full lips and high cheekbones that some people pay thousands of dollars to get.

Pregnancy can bring on a few challenges in skin, hair, and nails. And since it's harder for us to find the products that work for us, the last thing we need is a hormonal change that throws our usual program out the window.

With the help of hundreds of other black women, a hair stylist, and the noted dermatologist Dr. Susan C. Taylor, M.D.—author of *Brown Skin: Dr. Taylor's Prescription for Flawless, Skin, Hair and Nails* and director of the Skin of Color Center at Saint Luke's—Roosevelt Hospital in New York City—here are some survival tips for making the most of the beautiful you. Get your glow on!

SKIN

Problem
I've got acne. It's like I am a teenager all over again.

The Fix
It's those hormones. You may notice small pimples, blackheads, whiteheads, or larger spots on your face and body. Dr. Taylor's advice: "There are a few prescription or over the counter products that can be safely used during pregnancy or while nursing. Get your doctor's permission first, but she might approve use of benzoyl peroxide or salicylic acid. Both of these come in cleansers, creams, gels, or lotions, and are typically applied twice daily and require six weeks to have a positive effect on the skin. If your doctor won't give you the OK for these products, concentrate on

cleansing your skin properly twice a day. Avoid rubbing or scrubbing or any harsh products. Also, no picking or squeezing. You can try getting facials every few weeks, which can help prevent the follicles or pores from becoming plugged." Dr. Taylor's other tips include removing all makeup before bed, avoiding oily or greasy hair products, and wearing your hair off your face.

Problem

My skin is getting darker.

The Fix

An increase in hormone levels can stimulate your pigment-producing cells and cause hyperpigmentation in various areas, including the upper arms, thighs, genital area, and abdomen. Dr. Taylor says skin darkening is a common condition that occurs in nine out of ten pregnancies. In her book *Brown Skin*, she says, "On sun exposed areas of the skin, such as the arms and legs, apply a sunscreen with SPF 15 daily to prevent the sun from making any hyperpigmentation worse. Wear sunhats and stay out of direct sunlight. Because the discoloration stems from pregnancy hormones, it will most likely subside on its own within a few months after you give birth." You can also consider using products containing soy like Aveeno Positively Radiant, since soy has been demonstrated to even skin tone, according to Dr. Taylor.

Problem

My skin is so dry and itchy.

The Fix

Dr. Taylor advises limiting baths and showers to five minutes and using mild cleansers, such as Aveeno products, Cetaphil, and Dove. You can also use a thicker moisturizer, like Aquaphor, Eucerin Plus, or cocoa butter and shea butter. Vitamin E is another favorite, but Dr. Taylor warns that some people are allergic.

As your belly grows, the uterus presses down on the liver, causing secretions that could make the skin itch. Most antihistamines are not safe during pregnancy, but ask your doctor about Benadryl, or try a nonmedical alternative like Aveeno Oatmeal Bath, Dr. Taylor says. Another tip: Put your favorite moisturizer in the fridge before applying for a supercool and soothing experience. Another must-try is Bella Mama's Belly Oil, with lavender and neroli to combat the itchies.

Problem
I have a rash. Is it harmful?

The Fix
If you have a location rash on the abdomen, thighs, or chest, call your doctor right away, says Dr. Taylor, as this may indicate a serious condition. Any rashes that have pus or drainage, are bright red or warm to the touch, or have blisters or bumps with fluid in them are also red flags to call your doctor.

Problem
I'm sweating all the time.

The Fix
Wash with a deodorant soap, such as Lever 2000, and wear light-colored clothing made from breathable fabrics like cotton. Women, now with larger breasts, often find themselves sweating underneath their boobies. Dr. Taylor says that's the perfect place—moist and dark—for a yeast or fungal infection to occur. She recommends using a light dusting of unscented powder there and in other fold areas of the upper body. Wear only cotton bras, wash them regularly, and remove them at the end of the day to air out the area.

Problem
I have the "mask of pregnancy." What can I do?

The Fix

Melasma is a distressing pregnancy by-product and is characterized by light or dark brown patches on central facial areas like the forehead, cheeks, and nose or on the lower part of the face. Sunscreen, sunscreen, sunscreen, should be your mantra, says Dr. Taylor. She suggests avoiding the sun at all costs, since sunlight can further darkening, especially during summer, spring, and fall months. Apply SPF 45 daily and reapply every two hours or so. Dr. Taylor recommends one with zinc oxide or titanium dioxide, or both. You should also use a foundation with sunscreen. If the areas are very dark, try DermaBlend or CoverMark. Be aware that melasma may not go away on its own after delivery; you may have to seek treatment.

Problem

I've got more moles than ever before.

The Fix

Pregnancy hormones can cause all sorts of new skin growths on your face and body, from moles and skin tags to freckles. Moles that you already have may grow in size or get darker, and this is quite normal. However, Dr. Taylor says you should keep an eye on these developments since sudden changes in moles can also be a sign of skin cancer. "If a mole looks different from other moles on your body, grows larger than the diameter of a pencil eraser, or begins to itch, hurt, or bleed, see your dermatologist," Dr. Taylor says. Any normal moles can be easily removed after pregnancy by a dermatologist.

Problem

My facial hair is out of control.

The Fix

It's a pregnancy condition known as hirsutism. Dr. Taylor says that if the hair doesn't bother you, leave it alone. If you feel self-conscious, remove it by waxing, shaving, plucking, or threading. Do not use depilatories during pregnancy. But Dr. Taylor says laser hair removal is safe since it uses a light, not radiation.

Dr. Taylor's Best Pregnancy Skin Care Tips

1. If your skin is oilier, wash it more often, even two to three times a day. Use a foaming cleanser or oil-balancing soap, like Cetaphil Antibacterial Soap or Neutrogena Facial Cleanser Bar. If your skin is still oily after cleansing, apply an alcohol-free toner or astringent, and use it regularly.
2. Exfoliate. Since your skin may be particularly oily now, try exfoliating once a week or monthly with a mild clay or mud mask designed for oily skin.
3. Do not use any products or acne medications with vitamin A (such as retinol); these are not proven to be safe for pregnant women.

HAIR

Problem
Is it safe to relax my hair during pregnancy?

The Fix
There is no evidence that chemical processing in the form of relaxers or hair coloring has any effect on a developing fetus. Small amounts of these chemicals may find their way into the bloodstream, but at inconsequential levels. Some doctors recommend avoiding these processes in the first trimester when the fetus's organs are forming, just to be on the safe side. If you don't want to risk it at any point in your pregnancy, don't stop relaxing your hair cold turkey; this can cause damage to your hair, says Daria Wright, a New York–based hair care specialist. "Your stylist can determine what's best for your hair type and texture. Just as you go to your doctor for advice on other aspects of your pregnancy, you should

see a professional stylist about your hair," she says. Dr. Taylor suggests having one chemical treatment during the second or third trimester of your pregnancy.

Problem
What type of hair care routine is best for pregnancy?

The Fix
"You should wash and condition your hair weekly," advises Daria. "Use a conditioning shampoo for relaxed or curly hair texture. Avoid clear shampoos that have a glycerin base that strips the hair, but use a thick, creamy shampoo, followed by a detangling conditioner." Daria says we should cut out the volcano-hot blow dryers and the heat styling tools as well. "If your hair is not freshly shampooed, you shouldn't use heat styling. When your hair is just washed, there is moisture in it, but by the next day that moisture is gone so heat styling just dries it out more. It's like adding more heat to parched grass—your hair is just going to break off," she warns.

Problem
My hair texture changed.

The Fix
"This is the number one reason why you should not let your sister, girlfriend, cousin, or husband do your relaxer during pregnancy. When the hormones and oil secretions of pregnancy change your hair texture, your relaxer may not 'take' as well or it may burn you. A trained professional who knows you and your hair can tell how the texture has changed and make some adjustments in your chemical applications, perhaps a milder relaxer for a longer time or a stronger relaxer for a shorter time, but a trained hair professional can tell you this," says Daria. In addition to change in hair texture, Daria says, your scalp sensitivity can change too.

Problem

How can I camouflage my puffy face and spreading nose?

The Fix

The trick is to avoid extremes, Daria says—not pulling your hair all the way back or combing it forward into the face. "You want to create the illusion of up and out by having hair around the face. Add face framing curls or layers with height and width up and around the face to draw attention to your hair."

Problem

I'm sweating so much more. How can I protect my hair?

The Fix

Excessive perspiration, particularly at night, can wreak havoc on the hair. Daria recommends tying the hair down at night with a silk scarf to absorb the moisture. You can sit under a cool dryer in the morning, with the scarf still on, and this can help prevent matting or tangles. Perspiration can also lead to yucky, flaky buildup in the hair and along the hairline. "Some women see flakes and think they should add grease, but that's just making the matter worse. The key is washing more frequently—weekly," according to Daria.

Problem

I don't have time like I used to. I need a low-maintenance do for this pregnancy.

The Fix

The key to low-maintenance hair styling is the perfect haircut. "A good haircut is your foundation. If you are working too hard to style your hair, then you probably don't have a good haircut. Get yourself a good cut that works for your hair type, your face shape, and your lifestyle," advises Daria. The bob is a classic favorite among the low-maintenance crew. It looks good if you curl it and looks good if you don't. "It's very versatile too. You can wet set it for a completely different look," Daria says. If you want to go short, here's a caveat: supershort hairstyles à la Halle Berry are deceptively high maintenance and require a lot of trimming and shape-ups. If you want to go short, Daria recommends going short and natural, and just wash and go.

NAILS

Problem
My nails are weak and brittle.

The Fix
Weak, brittle nails that chip easily can be a sign of a vitamin deficiency, so you might want to mention it to your doctor. Here's Dr. Taylor's take on what to do: Simplify your nail care routine during pregnancy. Keep nails clipped regularly and file them gently. Massage a good hand lotion (Cetaphil, Neutrogena, Eucerin) directly onto the nail plate four times daily. Avoid "wet work" and water, which can further dry the nails. Nail polish and remover can actually further weaken your nails, so save the polish for special occasions. Acrylic nails are safe if applied in a well-ventilated place and if the technician is not cutting the cuticle skin around the nail plate. That can make weak nails worse. A Mocha favorite for rejuvenating dry nails is Creative Nail Solar Oil, infused with jojoba oil, rice bran, and vitamin E.

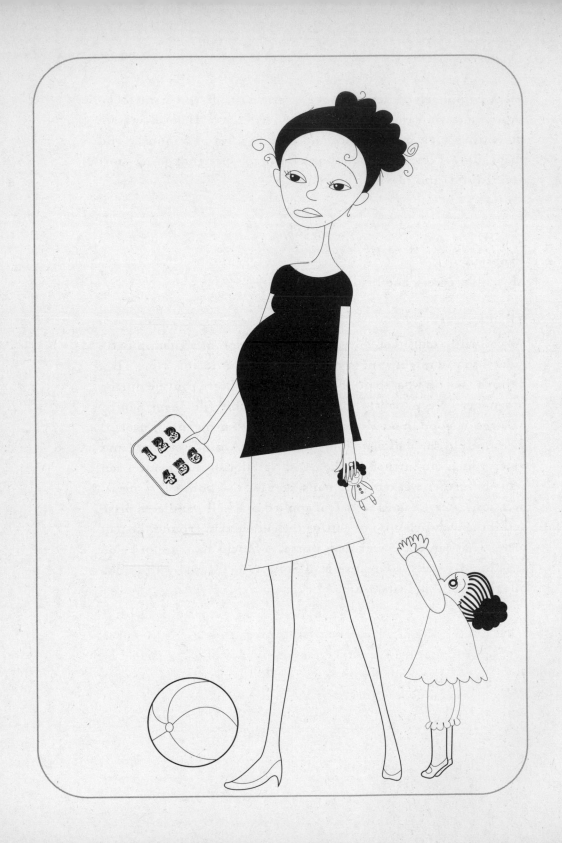

11

Back for More

PREGNANCY THE SECOND TIME AROUND

Your first pregnancy gets all the attention. When you're pregnant the second time, people give you the "Been there, done that," kind of vibe. Or, they reason, you should know the ropes because you've had a baby already. But having your second, third, or fiftieth pregnancy can bring on new feelings and fears. On the one hand, you know what pregnancy and delivery are like, but you may be worried because everybody and her mama say that "no two pregnancies are the same." This is true. In fact, the streets of mommyhood are littered with stories of the old bait and switch of pregnancies. That's when you have the most picture perfect, ideal, no-morning-sickness-no-vomiting-no-swollen-feet pregnancy, followed by a twenty-minute labor, two quick pushes, and not a stretch mark to be found. And then your second pregnancy is completely, totally, and utterly *not* like the first.

I'm speaking from experience. I had an enviable first pregnancy: Never vomited. My skin glowed. I gained the recommended weight. No swelling. I was dancing at a dinner party three days before I went into labor. My water broke while I was actually in my doctor's office, and exactly on my due date. That gave me enough time to stop at the Wendy's drive-through for a light snack of chicken nuggets before heading to the hospital. I was ridiculously calm and prepared. Okay, I couldn't dilate beyond eight centimeters, and I had to have a C-section. But in the end, I had a beautiful, healthy, eight-pound, four-ounce little girl. And, not a stretch mark to be found. It's a beautiful story, I know, a simple story. But then came my second pregnancy. Before I share that tale (and, yes, I was the victim of the ole bait and switch), let me say this: No pregnancy is exactly like the first. There will be a few mental and physical surprises. A second or third pregnancy has its own set of challenges.

Remember: in your first pregnancy, you had all that time to pamper yourself with manicures and pedicures, maybe a few pregnancy massages or a prenatal aerobics class here and there? Remember going home from work and putting your feet up (even if it was for that split second before you started a million other things!)? The problem is, you now have a little person waiting for you when you get home. And whether that child is one year old or nine years old, he still needs you. That little person still demands and expects the same amount of attention and energy you gave him before you were pregnant. In your first pregnancy, you may have had time to look after yourself and spend hours shopping and reserved for planning and personal reflection. But with all that is going on now, you may not have the same amount of time to devote to your pregnancy. As a result, your good eating habits may slack off, you may have less time to find cute clothes, your feelings about your appearance may waver, and you may be neglecting yourself even more than before. It's harder to get that extra rest when small hands are tugging on you to wake up. It's harder to sleep longer hours when you have a small being jumping, rolling, screaming, and/or still sleeping in your bed. And remember how everyone fawned over you with that first pregnancy—the joy, the attention, the two-hundred-person baby shower, and thirty-six diaper Genies— well, things just may be a little different this time. Let me tell you how.

First of all, prepare yourself that the reaction of your friends and family may not be as excited as it was before, especially if there's only been a short time since your first child. Throughout my second pregnancy, even strangers walked up to me and felt the need to comment about the spacing of my children. When I would tell them that my first was four years old, they would feel a need to say things like "Oh, that's a good gap" or "Good for you!" as if I needed commendation or cared what they thought about my reproductive time line. But as you know, strangers say the darnedest things to pregnant women. My girlfriend Isabel from Los Angeles recalls the dirty looks from old ladies as she walked around pregnant with her fifteen-month-old son in tow. Things can be worse if you already have more than one child. One friend with three kids would make sure she looked supertidy and her wedding rings were prominently displayed when she was pregnant for fear that she would be looked upon by old judgmental ladies as a welfare case.

The strangest reaction may even be from your partner. Lots of moms said their partner was less interested in the second pregnancy. Also, sometimes men feel an additional financial burden and anxiety with more than one child. I'm sure my husband did. Even though I was always working, one baby seemed manageable and two seemed more challenging. I think having two or more kids always involves the inevitable challenge of whether it's worth it (not just financially) for the woman to continue working or to stay home with the kids.

I remember my second pregnancy as nine months of guilt. I felt guilty that I didn't have the time to eat the way I did with the first.

I felt guilty that I wasn't reading and talking to the baby as often as I did with my first. With my first baby, I could easily recite what body part was developing in a given week. In my next pregnancy, I had trouble keeping tabs on how many weeks pregnant I was. First time around, I knew the right food to eat at that time to support that developing body part (Oh, it's a crucial week for the brain; let me load up on salmon and some omega-3 fatty acids!). At the next go-around, it was a personal challenge to take my prenatal vitamins every day. I found myself constantly apologizing to my unborn child for not being able to do more, eat more, talk more, and give more.

You may have similar feelings. You may even feel emotionally distant from this pregnancy. This is normal. My best advice is to devote five to ten minutes every day to thinking only about and planning for the coming baby—even if that means taking some time before going to sleep. Try to be as organized as possible to allow for this time and to avoid that always rushing feeling.

This may sound silly, but I worried that my second baby would be a bit of a letdown and that I couldn't possibly love it as much as my firstborn. I mean, my daughter is so beautiful, strong, and smart, and she is a constant reminder of a very significant accomplishment in my life. I still like to watch her sleep and I still get all teary-eyed. How could anyone else measure up to the wonder of that! I felt so blessed to have my daughter, I wondered whether having another would be pressing my luck. Then I felt guilty that I had such mixed feelings about the pregnancy. If you're thinking the same way, don't. It's perfectly normal to be sad to give up something you've treasured, such as the bond with an only child. And since your first child is here right now and the new baby isn't yet, it only makes sense that your feelings for the first child are stronger. Try just to acknowledge this reality to yourself without feeling bad about it. Of course, since having my precious baby boy, I now realize that each baby will amaze you with his or her own talents and characteristics, and that a mother's love is boundless.

There's plenty to go around. So don't worry. Most of all, take comfort in knowing that these confusing feelings are shared by thousands of women.

Taking childbirth classes again may also help increase the emotional involvement and attachment to the pregnancy. I absorbed a lot more the second time, when I was less anxious and neurotic and my brain wasn't overloaded with all the new things I'd read from millions of pregnancy books. A lot of other second timers felt they learned more because they were open to more possibilities, knowing that the path of labor is not etched in stone. Plus, it was set aside time to be with my husband and think about the baby.

This may also be a good time to toss out any old ideas about your body changes during pregnancy. First of all, you begin to show a lot sooner. My tummy started poking out the minute I peed on the stick. I'm sure I was no more than eight hours pregnant and somebody on the street was like "Oh, when are you due?" There was one particularly annoying clerk at the deli near my office. Here I was trying to be incogNegro about the pregnancy. I hadn't even told the boss yet and was grabbing lunch with a coworker. As I'm paying for my meal, the loud-mouthed cashier is like "You're pregnant, right?" She was apparently the newly crowned leader of the career and self-esteem destruction movement, and I just stood there with jaw dropped. "Yeah, I can tell from your stomach. What are you? Three months?" she continued, solidifying her position as captain of the pregnancy patrol squad. I was absolutely mortified and vehemently denied it all the way, cracking jokes about being bloated and saying that getting fat is still a constitutional right and basic American freedom. Then I blamed the weight gain on my job. It was a mess. I was now so paranoid, I walked around the office every day thereafter holding a number of files in front of my stomach, as a camouflage. And I don't even need files for my kind of work. Of course, after all of my subterfuge (files, blazers, shawls, arms folded in front of me, sitting down immediately when I entered someone's office) to delay telling my boss, when I did finally muster up the courage to share the news, he looked me in the eye and said, "Really? When are you due? You aren't even showing yet." Typical male, God bless 'em. But I was indeed showing early. And you probably will, too, since the previous stretching of your stomach muscles means that there's little resistance left and your tummy pokes out sooner.

You may also find that you have a lot of the sensations of pulling, tugging, and expanding about a month sooner than in your first pregnancy. This is because the uterus is less likely to give way for stretching. There are a few benefits to this stubborn uterus; for instance, you will also recognize fetal movements about a month earlier as well. Being a multipara (having more than one child) could also mean frequent and possibly more painful Braxton-Hicks contractions, especially toward the end of the pregnancy. Mine were so painful I was convinced this had to be labor, but every trip to the doctor showed zip, nada, nothing, on the dilatation front.

For Lavania from Greensboro, North Carolina, the second pregnancy was a fashion challenge. "I had no time to shop and find the kinds of nice things that made me feel good about being pregnant," she says. As it has for other women, less time for shopping and pampering had a direct effect on the way she felt about her body, which in turn affected her attitude and overall happy quotient during the pregnancy. "I didn't have the same head-up-high swagger," says Lavania. Make an earnest effort to "Do You" and find some feel-good activities.

Somehow, somewhere, find a moment to exhale. When people say that having two children is nothing like having one, they are telling you the gospel truth.

Mocha Mix: What the Sisters Say . . . About the Second Time Around

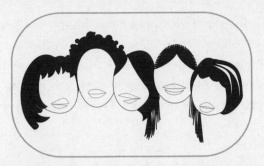

The first pregnancy I did my prenatal aerobics, monitored my protein and calcium intake on a daily basis, read absolutely everything in print on pregnancy, and rocked my high heel shoes to the end. My second pregnancy was reduced to one word—flats. There was no more time for prenatal aerobics, and I put on so much more weight in comparison that my feet were killing me. With my first, I didn't have to wear maternity clothes until I was about six months along. The second time, I broke them out around four months. I was definitely a victim of the good ole bait and switch. —DENISE, MANASSUS, VIRGINIA

I felt so guilty. Toward the end, the doctor said I couldn't pick up my older son anymore. It was horrible. I had this continual pull between the baby that was here and the one that was on the way. —STEPHANIE, BROOKLYN, NEW YORK

There was a lot more financial anxiety. Day care for two kids? College for two kids? It was like, oh my God! How are we going to do this? —REESE, DAYTON, OHIO

I had two completely opposite experiences. With my first my hair grew a lot; with the second one it didn't. I had terrible swelling of the feet and hands with my first child, but with my second—nothing. After having a boy at first, I figured it was a girl because it was such a different experience. But I have two boys, so different pregnancies don't always mean different genders. —PAMELA, NEW ORLEANS

My last child is seventeen years old. Being pregnant now is like starting all over from scratch and I couldn't feel happier. —DEBBIE, LOS ANGELES

When people saw that I was pregnant and I had a one-year-old, even strangers would ask me, "Did you plan it?" or pat my back and say, "You're very brave." It was really hard to deal with insensitive comments and sometimes I just wanted to stay home and avoid anyplace where people might look at me funny or say something stupid. —DEBRA, CHARLOTTE, NORTH CAROLINA

I felt much more in control with my first pregnancy. Before, if I needed to sleep all day, I could. Nobody was pulling on me to get up and go feed them. It's been a war to care for myself and care for my son. I'm trying to give my son some time before the baby comes, but I also have to take care of myself. —IVY, SAINT LOUIS, MISSOURI

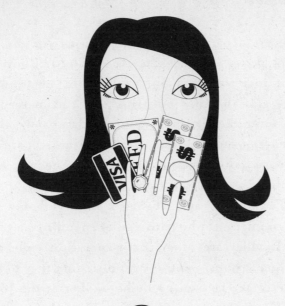

12

Mocha Money

THE NINE-MONTH GUIDE
TO FABULOUS FINANCES

You may have Manolos and a Marc Jacobs bag, but do you have moola in the bank? Let's face it: most black people are big on spending, and not so big on saving. Not that we're alone; the national savings rates are at all-time lows. But you know how we do; we have a Lexus with spinning rims but we still pay rent. Some of us confuse the term *assets* with the garments that cover our asses.

As beneficiaries of higher education and improved job opportunities, we are a part of the generation of African Americans whose buying power is expected to exceed $920 billion by 2008, a 189 percent increase from $316 billion in spending power in 1990. This gain handily outstrips the 128 percent expected increase in white buying power. But unfortunately, those bigger paychecks haven't automatically produced more confidence and savvy to manage money and turn it into sustained wealth.

One problem is often an overemphasis on conspicuous consumption. Economists say the behavior mimics that of other first-generation immigrants who have similar spending patterns. "Black professionals today are often first-generation college graduates who, like other groups, want to symbolize that they have arrived," explains Roderick Harrison, a demographer at the Joint Center for Political and Economic Studies. This plays right into the thinking in many professional circles: "If you want to achieve something, you have to act as if you already have it." Many of us translate that into "If you want to be financially successful, you must spend as if you already are." Therefore, our focus is on creating the image of success, by throwing money into depreciating assets like cars, clothes, and gadgets, but not building any real wealth. A study by the Consumer Federation of America and BET shows that while blacks are making more money, they aren't as quick to save or invest it. Black net wealth on average equals about $15,500 compared to the average $71,700 of net wealth accumulated by other Americans.

For most of us, talking about the stock market and investments is not typical dinner table conversation. In general, our cultural association with money has been "making ends meet," or it is a topic just for "grown folks."

Also race plays a part. Because African American women have a lot more to battle against and contend with in the fight for a healthy sense of self in this society, they often have a more difficult time in establishing good financial habits. Meanwhile, studies prove that blacks with similar credit profiles to whites still pay more for auto loans, home loans, and insurance. That means a greater portion of our income goes to current expenses, with less left for saving.

Yet as black women, we are still making strides. In a recent survey by a financial institution, 85 percent of African American women feel they are doing better financially now than they were twenty years ago. In fact, statistics from the Census Bureau show our median personal income increased nearly 75 percent between 1981 and 2001. That's heartening news.

When Sabrina, a curly-haired thirty-five-year-old earning $85,000 a year became pregnant, it brought a new set of financial worries. She had recently reduced her debt level from $7,000 to just over $3,000—an impressive accomplishment. She was saving about 3 percent of her annual income in the company 401(K) and was researching alternative investments like individual retirement accounts (IRAs). But getting a hold on your finances for yourself is daunting enough without the fear of having to provide for another human being. At some point, most of us have shifted into what I call *Good Times* money management mode. That's when an excessive shopping splurge leaves you with about twenty dollars till payday, and you sit around saying, "Damn, damn, damn," like Florida Evans of *Good Times,* and promising you'll never spend like that again. Of course, anyone in this situation probably knows the one spot near their job to eat for three bucks or slides the brown bag lunch into the briefcase for a few days. But having financial responsibility for a helpless little being is a bit more challenging. Sabrina was terrified of not being able to provide financially for her child. The first step is taking control of your mind and heart— changing your attitude about spending and shifting your focus to your child. Being a parent is nothing but perfecting the art of self-sacrifice, and this is a good time to start. Think of this nine-month plan as a journey and an investment in yourself and in your baby's financial future.

From the time you pee on the stick and that blue line appears, your life is forever changed. Your thinking must change, your habits must change, and your priorities must change. Just as eating the proper diet helps produce a healthy baby, changing your financial habits can yield positive financial fruit—like a debt-free life, money to invest in your and your child's future, and financial peace of mind.

This is not always easy. Many of us are financially tied to our jobs. Yet we may have envisioned staying home with our children and not returning to work right away. My mother never worked until we were school age, though I recall my father working two jobs at times—this was very important for both of them. Her presence every day was a defining element of the kind of mother I wanted to be. When I was pregnant with my first child, I was completing my master's degree via a fellowship at Columbia University and living off a fairly decent stipend. But with my baby due soon after classes, the thought of having to return to work a few months later left me paralyzed with fear.

After the panic, I created a three-step plan and dived in. One night, around my fourth month of pregnancy, I sat at my dining room table with a pen and a legal size pad.

Step one: I brainstormed and jotted down all of my qualifications and skills: undergraduate journalism degree from NYU, graduate journalism degree from Columbia, completed the New York State requirements for a secondary English education teacher, previous teaching experience. I dug deep, trying to remember everything I had done in my career: doing TV and radio interviews, editing Web sites and business plans for friends, and giving my entrepreneur buddies tips on how to drum up some press coverage.

Step two: I wrote down all the possible things I could do to earn money without going to work: freelancing as a journalist, being a media consultant, tutoring, part-time teaching at a private school, conducting writing workshops, editing business plans for a fee.

Step three: I worked the phones. I called nearly everyone I knew on a professional and personal basis and explained my situation and my desire to stay at home with my baby. I asked them to think of one or two people who might be able to help me.

As a result of this plan, a Wall Street investment banker who reviews hundreds of business plans a week said he could refer clients whose plans needed a bit more polish to me for advice and editing. A former editor at a previous job had recently helped launch a well-funded new magazine and needed freelancers. I jumped in. Another friend convinced his small company that they needed a media strategist and I was the perfect person for the job—given the going rates for media consultants and my extensive experience as a journalist I simply charged $500 less than the going rate and landed a six-month contract. The $3,000 monthly fee more than covered my expenses. My goal was to work from home for nine months. I ended up being at home with my daughter for two and a half years.

The work from my former editor helped me buy a reliable late model car for cash, leaving me free of a monthly car note and lowering my insurance premiums. We lived in a spacious three-bedroom apartment in Rosedale, Queens, and I willingly paid teenagers from my congregation to sit with my daughter for a few hours after school while I holed up in my home office to work.

To be honest, I have never worked so hard in all of my life. The hustle of freelancing, managing the lag time between submission and payments, along with the late and/or sleepless nights was overwhelming at times. Many times, I would put my daughter to bed and work all night until she woke up. But being there when she first sat up, rolled over, waved bye-bye, said "Hi," and reached other developmental milestones were the most fulfilling moments of my life. I've met other moms who did mystery shopping (go to a retail location as a customer and evaluate service, merchandise, or product distribution for that company) or started a small business. My friend Janelle, an administrative assistant with some serious typing skills, started her own word processing service catering to small businesses in her area.

I know this is not possible for everyone. But I have helped other pregnant women to use their pregnancy time to reduce expenses and to change their spending habits so that when baby arrives, they have more financial freedom to work less and mother more. Most importantly, we have to learn to trust ourselves. Many of us are chained to our "golden handcuffs" or paychecks. I know I was. The thought of not getting a paycheck every two weeks produced sheer terror. "How in the world do people live without direct deposit?" I would say to my prepregnancy self, waiting at the ATM at 9:00 A.M. on payday just to get some money. But I focused on the kind of mother I wanted to be for my child, and what ultimately would be in my baby's best interest, and then I set a reasonable time frame. If it wasn't working in four months, it was time to hit the bricks and find a job.

The main point is to develop a plan. So many times, as black people, we tend to drive by the seat of our pants. Studies show the majority of us don't plan for retirement, we don't plan for college savings, and we don't plan a budget. But straightening out your finances during pregnancy is all about a plan. Whoever said a failure to plan is a plan to fail was definitely right on point.

Even if you don't want to extend your maternity leave or having money while on leave is not a problem for you, there are still things that you need to do to prepare financially for your child. It's funny how we focus on the retail preparation for our children— buying this and that—but don't spend a minute thinking about how to childproof their financial future. Or we're too caught up in making ends meet now to think about the future. But as a parent, you have an obligation to take care of your baby in every way possible. That includes making sure that regardless of what happens to you, your child will be financially okay. These are things you need to do now, before baby arrives and you barely have the time to shower and get dressed every day.

The first step in any financial plan is self-evaluation: recognizing your desires and goals. Ask yourself whether staying home beyond your company maternity leave is important to you. For some, giving up or interrupting a career takes something away from their self-identity, and they want to get right back to work. We are not preprogrammed with the same vision of motherhood, and no one should judge another for a choice to work or stay at home. But returning to work immediately after the standard leave should be a choice, not something you are forced to do right away. I've met loads of women who said, "I didn't have a choice but to return to work," and sometimes this is absolutely true. Other times, there may be some ways at least to *delay* your return to work, especially since many companies are now offering some component of an unpaid leave to mothers.

Ask yourself, What are my spending habits and how may these be detrimental to my goals? Let's trim the fat and create the worst-case scenario by identifying the least amount of money you can get by on during any given month. Then we can use strategies and tools to slash costs and release hidden cash.

The final part of the preparation plan involves some specific financial planning strategies that all pregnant women should undertake. These include assessing your life insurance, starting a college fund, creating a will, and developing a systematic savings plan.

So let's get started.

The First Trimester

Month One

Self-Evaluation: Take thirty minutes a week for three weeks to brainstorm and revise a list of your personal and financial goals on the way to motherhood. Is taking a romantic or relaxing trip to the Caribbean (a babymoon, as it's called) before you take on the role of mother important to you? Write it down. Find your motivation. Is reducing expenses so you can stay at home beyond your paid company maternity leave important? Write it down. Be specific about how many months you would like to extend your leave. Categorize goals in the following areas: financial, emotional, spiritual, intellectual, professional, and physical, if applicable. Having a clear vision of what you want is critical.

Several motivational speakers, including Dr. Dennis Kimbro,

author of the national bestseller *Think and Grow Rich: A Black Choice*, suggest the need for clearly defined goals that are visible for consistent reinforcement. I don't know whether it really works for everybody. But I do know that putting my goals on a large posterboard in my bedroom, instead of tucked away in a notebook, kept me focused and motivated. Every day when I rose I saw them, thought about them, and tried to do at least one thing to put myself one step closer to those goals. Spend a few minutes each week focusing on your goals. Establish a routine to visualize, affirm, and meditate on your goals.

Action Plan: Review your life insurance policy. This is the most important thing any mom-to-be can do. It's up to you and your spouse to plan for the future. Life insurance can replace the lost income of a deceased spouse or partner and pay for future financial needs such as college education for the children. It may sound morbid, but you have to start thinking as a parent now. Even investments in the stock market are not a substitute for life insurance. And it's best to sort out your insurance before the second trimester, when medical conditions can develop, just in case an exam is needed. Plus, since you've been pricked and prodded so often and have peed in more than enough cups, your doctor knows more about you now than ever before, so a new exam may not even be necessary. Even if you are unmarried, talk to your child's father or build into any financial support agreements a provision for life insurance. This protects you and your child should something unforeseen happen to the father.

Here's a sobering fact: fewer than half of all American households have any life insurance beyond the usually inadequate amount provided by employers, according to A. M. Best & Co., an insurance rating company. There are numerous reasons life insurance is being ignored. People have grown more concerned about funding their retirement, so they're putting money into tax-favored retirement accounts instead of into life insurance premiums. At times, two-income families feel they can better weather the death of a spouse than a single-wage earner family. Nonetheless, owning adequate life insurance should remain an important part of your financial picture. You should make sure you have adequate life insurance before starting an investment program—even if that means paying the premiums with money that otherwise would have been invested.

Begin with your employer and make sure you are making full use of your benefits. Understand how much life insurance you and your spouse have. Company-provided coverage is usually not enough. You will typically need anywhere from five to ten times your annual income in life insurance coverage. Often an employer has an agreement with a specific insurance carrier that gives employees free consultations or discounted rates on spousal or other supplemental coverage. Then, work the Web. Hit up sites such as www.insure.com, www.underwriters.com, and www.acli.com to brush up on your insurance know-how; use calculators; view company comparisons; and even get quotes from a number of companies (see Appendix). Or for a free, computerized price quote service that helps you find up to six low-cost plans based on your age and health status, try one of these:

✳ Insurance Information: 800-472-5800
✳ SelectQuote: 800-343-1985
✳ InsuranceQuote services: 800-972-1104
✳ TermQuote: 800-444-8376

Most take payments directly from your bank account; that gives you one less bill to remember, and you'll really appreciate it as pregnancy brain sets in.

To figure out how much insurance you might need, consider your short-term needs (expenses, outstanding debts, and emergency expenses), long-term needs (housing payments), education (dependents' college tuition), family maintenance (child care, food, clothing, utility bills, insurance, and transportation), and assets such as savings, stocks, bonds, mutual funds, and other insurance.

Term insurance is the most cost-effective, simple, basic, and appropriate life insurance policy available for families with children. You pay a yearly premium for a set period (called a *term*, from one to thirty years), and if you die during this term, your survivors receive the full amount of your coverage. Here are a few guidelines. A good term policy should be:

✳ Automatically renewable for the duration of the term: During each year of a fifteen-year plan, you can renew regardless of your health. In a standard, inexpensive term plan, your premium will probably increase annually.

✳ Renewable for as long as you want: At the end of a fifteen-year term, you should have the option of renewing for another period (at higher rates), until age seventy.

✳ Convertible: A cash-value policy might make more sense when you're older. So look for a term policy that enables you to convert it to a cash-value plan—without a health exam—up to age sixty-five. Think about switching in your fifties, not before.

Consider disability insurance: If you are a primary breadwinner or a single mom, strongly consider increasing or obtaining disability insurance, which can cover a percentage of your salary if you become disabled and can't do your job. In most cases, your chance of becoming disabled is greater than your chance of dying while your child is young.

With these basic protections taken care of, you can now focus on your current financial predicament.

Month Two
Self-Evaluation: What three things am I willing to do to spend more time at home with my baby? What financial habits are preventing me from having greater financial success?

Action Plan: Get to know your cash flow. Now that we've taken care of the future, let's start tackling the present. Remember that the most important tenets of getting a grip on your finances is to set priorities and make choices. Some of those choices won't be easy and may require discipline, restraint, or even some self-aversion tactics. But you can do this. Remember that regardless of how society, the media, or anyone else portrays black women, we come from a long line of women who were extremely resourceful, were not necessarily well off, but managed to raise families (some large) and hold it down. Still, some of us may have some unhealthy ideas attached to money. Many women reading these words are blessed to be part of the new group of upwardly mobile women who have scaled corporate ladders and kicked down doors of opportunities. But those successes aren't automatically based on the skills and confidence to manage our money affairs. A lot of our sisterfriends who have it going on the job front may be subconsciously caught up in making themselves acceptable to a world or a workplace that doesn't show them much love. I see it all the time: expensive bags, expensive shoes, expensive clothes and hair, skin, and nail maintenance, all to look the part of success or perhaps subconsciously prove something to or impress white people. You may even be using expensive items to heal emotional wounds. Now, don't get me wrong: I believe in retail therapy, a sensible "treat" once in a while and an expensive splurge every now and again, but feel-good spending that piles on mounds of credit card debt or uses cash when there is no savings will never lead to anything but trouble.

Many of the sisters who did find themselves in financial trouble were too proud to get help or admit to a problem. Since they were viewed as "successful" or admired as an example to their family and friends (at least by all outward appearances), they were too ashamed to admit to a credit or spending problem. Others just couldn't turn off the ATM they had become to loved ones. Their need to "help" or be perceived as in a position to help pushed their credit score into the toilet and kept their bank account empty.

911 ALERT: If your finances are completely out of control and you don't think you'll get them organized before you give birth, get professional help! Contact an accountant or financial planner, or check out some of the free or low-cost debt counseling services available in your area (see Appendix). Ask a friend for a referral, and be sure to do a background check of any professional before sharing personal information or your money.

Regardless of your situation, everybody has a little bit (at the very least) of work to do.

Action Plan: Make a concise list of all of your income and expenditures (see Worksheet on page 286). This is known in the financial planning world as a cash flow analysis. You can't know what you're dealing with until you jot it all down. Write down all of your fixed bills, such as mortgage, car, insurance, or student loans; variable expenses, such as utilities, cell phone, car maintenance; as well as money spent on miscellaneous items such as coffee, lunch, movies, and manicures. You may want to pull out old receipts, bank statements, and credit card bills to see how much money goes on restaurants, clothes, gas, entertainment, and so forth. This will help you see where your money is going every month and where you can plug up the money holes. This exercise alone can be really eye opening. There's a lot of "I had no idea I was spending that much on . . ." as women go through this process. Then write down how much money you or you and your spouse earn every month, including income and any benefits or interest payments coming in. The bottom line is that if you are spending more than you earn, there's a problem that needs to be addressed. In order to save, you will have to learn to spend less than you earn. This may sound daunting, but before you break out in a cold sweat, you should realize that developing a flexible spending plan is not painful.

Let's look at what expenses can possibly be lowered. Are you spending a lot in any particular areas, say, shopping or, um, shopping? Don't feel bad. Recent estimates show that at least 5 percent of the population suffer from compulsive shopping problems. (Take a test to see whether this applies to you on page 285.) Are there any choices you can make, such as giving up restaurant outings twice a week, to help cut back? Can you live without cable for a while, or at least the expensive upgrades? Trust me: you'll be doing a lot more sleeping and retiring early now that you're pregnant. Start out small and implement one money-saving strategy a week. I'll get back to some more money-saving ideas in a minute, but for now I want you to focus on our goal here—trying to get you more time at home with that beautiful baby of yours.

So let's get back to the baby. What's your magic number? How many additional months of unpaid leave or part-time work do you want to take, or do you think it is reasonable to ask your boss for? If your company gives only three months of paid leave but offers more unpaid leave, you may want to add three months or more to your total leave. Talk about it with your husband or partner. He's going to have to make some sacrifices, too. Having a conversation about your shared parenting desires for your child and how much this means to you can help you both get your game face on to figure this out.

My friend Shelley from Camden, New Jersey, couldn't see how they could survive without her income, and she was apprehensive about even mentioning it to her husband because it seemed so unrealistic anyway, and she thought it would put extra pressure and stress on him. But they were able to work out a plan that let her stay home for two extra months after her paid leave ended.

This magic number serves as your joint goal. We now need to translate that number into a preliminary dollar figure. For instance, if your magic number is three months, and your family contribution or need from your income is $3,000 per month, then you will need about $9,000 saved up to stay home for three months. Either way, your goal for Month Two is to determine a magic number, trim all the excess fat out of your spending, and have a starting point for the amount of money you need to sock away to reach that goal.

Most families find they can live on about 80 percent or less of their monthly net income while on leave. Once you've got this amount in your head, divide it by the amount of months you have left. Don't forget to include the months of paid leave you have coming to you, and remember that not going to work can actually save you a bundle on transportation, lunch, dry cleaning, and clothing costs. My commuting costs run about three hundred dollars a month—just to get to work! So staying home automatically shaved those dollars off the budget and put them to use elsewhere.

Now, here are some more suggestions on reducing your expenses. And remember to be open to temporary situations that can help you reach your permanent goals:

Refinance your mortgage: For every $10,000 of your mortgage loan, a half percent difference in the interest rate saves you more than $40 a year or $3.40 a month in interest expense. That means that a $100,000 loan at 9½ percent refinanced to a lower 7½ percent saves $142 per month or $1,704 a year, for a total of $50,991 over the life of a thirty-year mortgage.

If you have built up equity in your home and are refinancing, you may be able to get cash out of your home to finance an extended leave or pay off some or all of your debts and free up some cash. In some cases, you can lower your mortgage payment and walk away debt free—a big win! But consider the pros and cons of tapping into your home's equity, especially if you plan on selling soon and may not be able to rebuild that equity before that time. Debbie and Lamar from Sacramento, California, did this. They refinanced their mortgage, tapping into some but not all of their home equity to pay off their credit cards and auto loans. When it was all over, they saved about $320 a month or $3,840 a year on their mortgage and now had no debt payments. That allowed them to save more money aggressively over the course of their pregnancy. Paying off all their debts bumped up their credit score, and they later applied for a low-interest credit card. With no debt and a good score, they easily received a $5,000 credit limit. That credit card was money to be used to help finance an extra three months off from work. The money they saved up during the pregnancy was applied to other monthly bills such as insurance and utilities. The credit card was used for groceries, gas, and other items. They never intended to pay that card off every month, but allowed it slowly to accumulate a balance, paying off a little more than the minimum every month. When Debbie returned to work and they were back to full financial throttle, they aggressively attacked that bill, getting it down to a zero balance in less than three months.

Cut your wheels: Jill and Carlos from Livonia, Michigan, decided one car would suffice for fifteen months (nine months of pregnancy, three months of paid leave, and three months of unpaid leave). They took the license plates off and put their newer car (the one with the higher premiums) in the garage to eliminate insurance payments. They saved $330 a month or $4,950 over the fifteen months by using only their less flashy older model vehicle, which was fully paid for.

You can also reduce your insurance costs by raising your deductible. Increasing your deductible from $200 to $500 can shave 15 to 30 percent off your collision and comprehensive coverage. Bumping it up to $1,000 could save up to 40 percent. While you have the insurance company on the phone, ask about all the discounts (car-alarm, low mileage, defensive driver courses) they offer, and see whether you qualify for any additional savings.

Check your connections: Look at where you can save with your long-distance phone, cell phone, and Internet bills. The Internet is bursting with sites that allow you to compare plans and utility providers in your area.

Brown-bag it: Can your take your own lunch to work at least one or two days a week? In some major metropolitan cities, lunches can easily cost $8 to $10 a day or up to $50 a week, or $200 a month. Do the math: saving $200 a month for 9 months = $1,800. Plus, you'll have more incentive to eat healthy since you prepare it and pack it yourself.

Coffee jar: Are you hooked on a $3 or $4 latte or one of those mochalatochinos? You can't do your caffeine thing anymore anyway, so try cutting out the overpriced decaf version as well. Water is so much better for you and could put an extra $80 a month back into your pocket.

Your crib: Not the one for your baby, the one where you live. Is it costing you an arm and a leg? Can you move to a less expensive apartment? If you have a one-bedroom, resist the urge to upgrade right away: babies rarely need or even use their own room in the first year.

If you're a single mom or your husband is really cool with your in-laws, is it possible to stay with family or relatives during your pregnancy and rent out your apartment on a short-term basis? If you have a spare room or own a house, can you rent out a room or basement to a trustworthy friend or highly recommended acquaintance for say, six months, or longer?

I was fortunate enough to be living in New York City in late 1999 at the turn of the millennium. With all the excitement about bringing in the new millennium in New York, there was a frenzied demand for accommodations for the truckloads of people who were piling into New York to go to Times Square. I was pregnant at the time and was planning on doing the quiet family thing. So I called a few realtors and hit a few Web sites and marketed my apartment as a possible New Year's accommodation that was available for a week or longer. With New York City hotel prices soaring to $350 a night and beyond, I made my place attractively priced at $100 and a realtor found a couple from the Midwest who were interested. They paid $1,000 for 10 nights! I just stocked up on toilet paper, soap, and some cheap linens (which I threw out, because you know how we are about strangers!) and packed up some valuables and photos in a box. To this day, I can't believe I actually got paid to chill at my folks' house eating my mom's home cooking every night and playing house guest while they completely fawned over me.

Of course, I don't have to tell you to be careful about who you let into your home. The streets are full of crazies and, even worse, nasty people who leave your place in a state. Realtors tend to do a good job of checking out a person's background, employment, credit history, and other credentials. But these days, even that is no guarantee.

THE SECOND TRIMESTER

Month Four

Self-Evaluation: Now that your household finances are lean, trim, and about as tight as Beyonce's butt, this is the trimester you can really pump up the savings and reduce debt.

With your energy levels returning, some women opt for a little overtime, once or twice a week, to add a few pennies to the coffers. Is there something else you can do for a little extra cash? This may be a good idea, if you don't push yourself too hard. Sondra, from Allentown, Pennsylvania, would eat at her desk and then take a power nap in her car during her official lunch hour whenever she planned to work a few hours overtime. Also, pack your snacks and water to keep your energy up and prevent dehydration.

Action Plan: Take your monthly savings goal and divide it by the number of paychecks you receive every month. That's how much you need to sock away from each pay period. Money that reaches your pocket has a slim chance of making it to the savings account. Set up some automatic deductions into a high-interest savings account. Most banks allow you to set the dates, so choose your paydays so the money goes before you have a chance to get at it. With your savings plan on autopilot, continue to reduce expenses, cut spending, and bank the extra cash. Here are some more ideas:

Become a cash queen: Spending is way too easy with all the debit cards and fifteen ATMs on every corner. Do yourself a favor: go to the ATM once and get your money for the week. Then put your debit and credit cards away. Lock 'em up. Have your husband, friend, or mother hide them from you. Live on a cash allowance for the week, and when it's gone, it's gone, until next week. My husband and I try to do this now because we realized all of those spontaneous trips to the ATM, along with the fees for using out-of-network banks, ate up our money. We get our cash allowance for the week and the debit cards get put away—okay, it's mine that has to be confiscated; my husband actually has the discipline not to go to the ATM.

Got stuff? Sell it! Have a garage sale to raise cash or put some clothes on consignment and use the proceeds to pay down debt.

Stay home: It sounds so simple, but imagine how much money you'll save by staying home and nesting. If your home is a cluttered mess, take some time to clear that clutter out of your living space. When your home is warm and inviting, you'll have less desire to leave it to spend more money.

Play bill collector: Have you lent money to friends, relatives, or play cousins and not seen one red cent since? Now is a good time to go collecting. You may have felt bad in the past for asking for the money (or felt bad that you had to ask, which is true), but with your new circumstances you've got the perfect excuse and people are certainly more sympathetic to your situation. When you call, play up your need to get prepared for the baby, and then let them know you want your money—yesterday!

While you're in collection mode, check with your former employers to see whether you left any 401(K) funds, pension assets, or stock options that are due you. Research your options for what to do with any unclaimed cash.

Month Five
Action Plan: Attack debt. If credit card and other debts are standing between you and extended time with your baby, you have two paths to take. If it's possible to pay off a high-interest or high-

minimum-payment card before you stop working, then you can aggressively pay down the debt, thereby freeing up cash to save and use elsewhere. Or some couples have chosen to continue making on-time regular payments on their credit cards, focus on spending less and saving more, and attack debt later when everyone is back at work. To them, the debt has been around long enough, and an extra six months or so is not going to kill anybody. I've seen both plans work well.

The only problem is that often a mom, even after an extended leave, decides she just doesn't want to go back to work anymore. Many times, even the most high-powered career woman is surprised that her desire to get back in the game is gone. But when looming debt is put off, and returning to work is already priced into the financial plan, you can still find yourself exactly where you didn't want to be—with no choice but to return to work. Even if you had six months or more at home, going back to a place you don't really want to be is painful. You and your partner should talk about what makes both of you most comfortable.

Until then and from this day forward, you have a new attitude about debt. Repeat after me: I will not create new debt! I will not create new debt! This is your mantra, your affirmation, your pledge, your words to live by from here on in. No matter what happens, what stroller or newfangled crib you see, you will not buy it on credit. You can't eliminate debt if you keep adding more—this is not rocket science. This is when you need to exercise discipline and to stay focused on your baby. For a few months, when I lost my discipline and struggled with bouts of spontaneous and continuous shopping, I took my treasured sonogram picture and folded it around my credit card. Every time I went to use the card, I saw my precious baby and remembered my goal of staying home longer. Eventually, I was able to take the credit card out of my bag altogether and give it to my husband to hide for me.

My friend put her credit card in a Ziploc bag filled with water and froze it. When she was debt free she had a few girlfriends over to share a champagne toast and watch the "plastic ice block" melt.

The thing was, Kenya was so happy with her cash-only existence and the feeling of not owing anyone or hiding from creditors, that when the credit card thawed, she cut it up that very night.

If you know you have a shopping problem, get your girlfriends and family to help. When you go a whole week and month without using a card, give yourself a small reward. Make it a challenge or a game, with plenty of little rewards along the way.

Student loans: Call your lender to see whether they will offer you forbearance or a deferment for a few months.

Debt consolidation: Consider a debt consolidation loan or a service that works with your creditors to reduce interest rates and offers one monthly payment. One caveat: some credit counseling services will appear on your credit report and possibly send a red flag to future lenders.

Month Six

Action Plan: Think ahead.

Child care: Child care costs are through the roof practically everywhere; but it's one area in which I don't believe in skimping. Don't ever go the cheapee route when it comes to who is looking after your baby. This trimester is a good time to use your energy to start investigating options and costs, especially in places where waiting lists for small babies are the norm.

Start a file: Keep your baby's papers in order from the very beginning, and you'll give her life a stable base. Include information on insurance benefits and savings and checking account details. After the birth, you can easily add the birth certificate and social security card.

Start a college fund: It's never too early to start a college fund, and even if you don't have enough money in your budget to start heavy-duty investing at this point, there are other options. When you start saving early, even a small amount like $10 a week can turn into a sizable pot by the time the college years approach.

Think about starting a 529 college savings plan. You can often start a plan for as little as $25. This investment account allows you to rack up money for your child's education and it grows tax-free. Uncle Sam won't tax your money when you take it out of the account as long as it's used for higher education—at any public or private accredited college or university in the country. Any family, regardless of income, can contribute, and there's a lifetime contribution maximum of about $290,000 (depending on your state). The 529 plans are administered by individual states, but you don't have to invest in the plan of your state. You can choose the state that best meets your needs, but keep in mind that a nonresident may not get the state tax benefits, may be charged higher commission rates, or may not have access to the full range of investment options.

The big plus of 529 plans is that the money is considered your asset, not your child's. That means that stash in a 529 plan has no bearing on your child's eligibility for financial aid, unlike most other college savings vehicles, which are viewed as an asset of the child's. And if your superstar child gets a full-tuition academic scholarship, the money can be transferred back to you tax-free and without penalty. The Internet is loaded with more information about 529s and your state's plan, so do a little research (see Appendix). A broker can set one up for you, but be mindful of hefty commissions that can eat up your returns in the early years. Be sure always to read the fine print about restrictions and penalties, and watch out for the annual maintenance fees and commissions.

Another concept that's gaining momentum are companies like Upromise and BabyMint. These companies have rebate programs that let you earn money (similarly to earning airline miles) for your child's education through purchases at certain stores. You just have to register your credit, debit, or drugstore cards (you can register grandma, grandpa, and auntie's cards, too), and when you shop at more than one hundred national stores, nine thousand restaurants, ten thousand hotels, and so on (in the case of UPromise), you earn a small percentage of your purchases, which goes into your account. The caps on the account mean you won't be able to foot the entire college bill, but you can make a dent.

Note: Any good financial planner will tell you that you should *not* save for college unless you already have a retirement savings plan in place. Save for your retirement first. There is no fallback plan for you. This may sound like selfishness or a page out of the tough love handbook, but in a worst-case scenario, your child can fund his college education the old-fashioned way—loans up the hilt and a Pell Grant. Trust me: it's no fun bragging about Johnny being debt-free at Harvard when you're living on social security pennies and eating sardines three nights a week.

THE THIRD TRIMESTER

Month Seven

Self-Evaluation: You're in the final stretch. Reward yourself for your hard work and financial sacrifices and take heart, knowing that you are starting new habits that put your financial future in better standing. Perhaps as you approach the final weeks of your pregnancy, your savings pot is not as fat as you would have liked. You may even have to shorten your planned pregnancy leave. This may be a bit disappointing, but you can make the best of it by trying to find a close, supportive, and dependable relative to help you with child care. Perhaps you can arrange to have child care near your workplace so you can pop in during lunch and break time to visit or even breast-feed.

Action Plan: Get showered.

Baby shower: Yep, a baby shower is part of your financial plan. Around this time you start itching to buy stuff for the nursery or some other baby gadgetry that you just don't need. Even if you resist most of the impulsive buys (what's the point of being pregnant without a few splurges!), the stuff you do actually need costs money. Before you go crazy, check with your friends about giving you a baby shower. Check with coworkers for a little office party as well. Don't be scurred or shamed. Go register your needs at a baby store and spread the word. If you're philosophically opposed to a registry (although I can't imagine why), give your closest friends or the shower organizer a wish list. Guests will likely ask the organizer about your needs, so make sure she's prepared.

Knowing you will have a baby shower eases some of the financial burden of buying all the stuff a baby needs. Wait until after the shower to make any major purchases. You'll probably be surprised by the generosity of your friends and relatives. You can also borrow many items from other moms—just be careful of older cribs and car seats as the safety guidelines for these change pretty often.

If you're far away from close friends and family (or your hormonal moodiness has isolated you from everyone), feel free to throw a "welcome to the world" party for your baby. Framing it this way takes the focus off you and shifts it to the baby. Who can resist getting a welcome gift for a new baby?

Now, how are you going to resist spending hours strolling down all the lanes at your local baby superstore? Or pointing and clicking your way to a pile of boxes delivered to your doorstep? Well, you have plenty of other work to do, my dear. It's the tough stuff, so buck up, but it is absolutely necessary.

Months Eight and Nine
Action Plan: Do the tough stuff.

A will: This may put a real damper on your pregnancy buzz, but these are the things a parent must think about. You need a will, no way around it. It basically lays out where your assets are to go if you die. It should also state who should take care of your child and his or her finances. Remember, people, godmother is not a legal designation; these things have to be laid out properly.

While you're at it, check the name of beneficiaries of retirement accounts such as any IRAs or 401(K)s you have. These may need to be updated now that you have a child of your own.

Durable power of attorney: Wills are good, but they aren't perfect. They cover you in case of death, but don't cover you if you're severely incapacitated. This is particularly important for single parents. If you have a stroke or an incapacitating illness, a will won't help sort out who will pay your bills, make deposits, arrange for your care, and look after your money. That is where a durable power of attorney comes in. A *regular power* of attorney gives another person legal authority to act on your behalf should you die. A *durable power of attorney* means that the person you have selected, your agent, will also act on your behalf if you are incapacitated whether or not a court deems you incapacitated. It is a simple, easy way to make sure your finances stay in the hands of a trusted person you choose. To create a durable power of attorney, the document must clearly use specific language according to your state's guidelines. For example, in most states, the document must say in substance that "this power of attorney shall not be affected by subsequent disability or incapacity."

To create a legally valid durable power of attorney, you need only to complete and sign a fill-in-the-blanks form that is a few pages long. Finding such a form may require a little legwork or an attorney. About a dozen states have their own forms published in the statute books. Go to a law library and look up *Durable Power of Attorney* in the index to the state statutes. Then type out a document, following the model form exactly. After you complete the form you must sign it in the presence of a notary public. In some states, a witness may be required. Note: Some banks and brokerages have their own such forms. To make sure your agent doesn't have any difficulty acting on your behalf, you may have to complete the bank's form as well as the general form.

Revocable trust with an incapacity clause: Sounds absolutely horrible, right? I know, but please stay with me: you need the best protection for your child. This mouthful of a document details how you want your finances handled if you become incapable of making these decisions for yourself. If you die, the trust becomes the blueprint for the way you want your finances to be managed. And if you happen to die when your child is a minor, the revocable trust takes care of the child's well-being and eliminates the need for your family to go through the process of probate guardianship.

This all sounds time-consuming and mentally taxing, but there are actually CD-ROM programs to help you draw up your own personalized documents based on the laws in your state. All of these documents will have to be notarized to go into effect. You can also hire an attorney who specializes in trusts (see Appendix). She should charge you a flat fee, depending on the amount of your assets. The more assets you have, the more expensive creating the trust is.

Durable powers of attorney for health care: This document details your wishes about how you want doctors to care for you if you become critically ill or require life support. You can usually get one from a hospital at no cost.

Whew! Congratulations, you've done the tough parent work of making sure everything is set up to take care of your family if you should die, become critically ill, or be incapacitated. Now you can get on with parenting, relieved to have your business in order. Since you've gone through the hard work of financially protecting your children and making the process legally binding, reward yourself. Reward yourself with what women all over the world do to make themselves feel better: talking.

Talk: Set aside time to have a talk with your partner about the financial aspects of raising your kids. We can spend a lot of time thinking about how you can "afford" children, but there are other aspects to child rearing: Will there be allowances? What types of gifts are permitted? Are you planning on public school or private school? How much should be spent on clothing for the child? Know your partner's financial philosophy about kids. My husband was raised on the basics, by a single mother who had six kids, so he couldn't always understand my definition of "necessary" spending on our children. Bridget, a brand-name-labelmeister from Mount Vernon, New York, hit a few road blocks with her husband when she took home BabyGap, baby Guess!, and Polo by Ralph Lauren and he proudly took home loads of "slightly irregular" baby clothes from Costco, the wholesale store. " 'Nobody notices that one leg is slightly shorter than the other,' he says; 'But I do,' " says Bridget. "And irregular is not good enough for my baby. It always led to an argument." Having a conversation about the financial rules of the house and future guidelines for the kids can help limit the drama down the road.

Set a good example: All of these preparations won't mean a hill of beans if you aren't a strong financial role model for your children. When you think about the values you want to instill as a parent, consider their financial savvy. What lesson is taught when we're swimming in credit card debt, living check to check, or have no real savings but drive luxury cars. Our job as a role model to our children includes money-smart principles. Our responsibility as black people is to break the cycle of having no real assets or substantial wealth to live on or to pass on to our children.

Now that you are truly a hot mocha mama—in mind, body, and wallet—may your journey in pregnancy and motherhood give you all the joy your heart and hands can hold.

SHOP TILL YOU DROP
Are You a Compulsive Shopper?

We all know a sister who's got more spending issues than *TV Guide*, but what if that sister is you? Worse yet, what if you don't know that it's you? Clinical tests prove compulsive spending is the leading cause of financial death. Left unchecked, this sort of spending has damaged relationships and ruined credit. It is a real disorder, complete with its own anonymous support group and 800 numbers.

Take this simple quiz to see whether you show signs of a compulsive spending habit. Be warned: this habit can easily transfer from shopping for yourself to shopping for baby.

If you answer yes to more than half of these questions, then you may have a problem. Consider distracting yourself with other activities, shopping only when someone else is with you, or destroying all credit cards except one for emergencies. You can also get help from organizations like Debtors Anonymous, which have meetings nationwide.

1. Are all of your credit cards maxed out?
2. Are you ducking debt collectors? Or is worry over debts making you lose sleep or affecting your work productivity?
3. Do you get cash from your credit card to pay for rent or food?
4. Do you leave packages in a car, the front closet, or your friend's house, to hide purchases from your partner?
5. Do you feel a need to shop rather than a desire to shop?
6. Do you have a sense of exhilaration when you shop and then feel guilty afterward?

The B Word—A Budget Worksheet

*B*udget doesn't have to be a dirty word. Use this simple worksheet to track your spending so you can figure out where your money is going and where you can make some changes. Do Parts One, Two, and Three focusing on the Current Spending column first to find out whether there's spare cash for saving or a little belt tightening to do. Then use the Revisions column to make some adjustments and plan your New Budget.

Part One: Calculate Your Monthly Income

Salary _____

Other Pay _____

Investment Income _____

Other Income _____

Total Monthly Income = _____

Part Two: Monthly Expenses

Expense	Current Spending	Revisions	New Budget
Rent or Mortgage			
Insurance			
Property Taxes			
Gas and Electric			
Water			
Telephone			
Groceries			
Eating Out (Include Coffee and Drinks)			

Car Payments			
Auto Insurance			
Gas			
Car Repairs and Maintenance			
Parking Fees			
Commuting/Transit			
Medical/Health Insurance			
Clothing			
Credit Card Payments			
Loan Payments			
Other Debt Payments			
Cable/Video/Movies			
Internet Access			
Subscriptions			
Hobbies and Sports			
Gym Membership			
Vacations			
Religious, Charitable Donations			
Laundry/Dry Cleaning			
Child Care			
School Fees			
Gifts			

Savings Account			
Emergency Fund			
Mutual Funds, Stocks, or Bonds			
Miscellaneous Expenses			
Total Monthly Expenses =			

Part Three: Shortage or Surplus

Total Monthly Income _____

Total Monthly Expenses _____

Monthly Surplus/Shortage = _____

Acknowledgments

They say no man is an island, and in like manner, no book is ever really a solo project. And so it is with this one. This book would not have been possible without the help, support, and sleep deprivation survival strategies of a host of friends, family, and colleagues.

First, I want to thank Jehovah God for giving me the strength "beyond what is normal" to complete this project, as I constantly saw your hand directing matters on my behalf. I want to thank my parents, Alma and James Seals, who have supported me from my first short story in the third grade until now, all along the way teaching me to reach for my dreams and believing in me even when I doubted myself. I am who I am because of you two. A special thanks to the rest of my family: my sister and brother-in-law, Katrina and Richard Ruiz; my brother, Jeffrey Seals; my great-grandmother, Helen Nurse; my auntie, Margretta Fairweather; my uncle, James Billy Jr.; and my nieces and nephews, Richard Jr., Autumn, Bria, and Jonathan.

To my Allers family across the pond in London, especially my mother-in-law, Elizabeth Allers—your life of perseverance and struggle teaches me that sometimes having less allows you to give more. To Pamela Alexander, thanks for being a shoulder to lean on, and to Deceilia Alexander, know that I'll never forget the love and care you showed me when others wouldn't. Thanks to the rest of my Allers crew: Dominick, Marion, Willston, Frances, Karen, Melissa, Richard, Denyce, Chloe, Naomi, Kaielle, Ciaran, Georgia, Junaelle, and Terrelle.

Where would I be without my sisterfriends? Sherese Shepard, Schalawn Warren, Donna Anderson, and Keiva Miller—girls, thanks for the laughs, the love, and the encouragement. Your friendship is truly treasured. Then there's my friend, Cora Daniels, who plays shy and talks tough, but together we redefined ourselves for ourselves, even when others were overlooking our talent. And I must acknowledge Sukkiim Cover and Sabrina Rote who took good care of my little darlings while I was tucked away writing.

Nicholas Roman Lewis, my agent extraordinaire—thank you for supporting me, keeping my neuroses in check, and generally watching my back. And to my editor, Dawn Davis—a true mocha mama herself, thank you for being passionate about this project and pushing me to make this book hot!

But this book really, really, really, wouldn't have happened without the countless women who shared their pregnancy stories—often with joy, sometimes in tears, but always with love and in the spirit of knowing that pregnancy and motherhood is the most beautiful privilege known to womankind. Thank you for making time in between morning sickness and midday snacks, or diaper changes and breastfeeding to share your journeys. I am forever grateful.

Last, but certainly not least, I want to thank my husband and my children. Joseph, we have been through so much together and I am extremely proud of what we have accomplished in life, love, and family. Thank you for warming my cold feet every night, even when I climbed into bed at 4 A.M after a writing spree, your creative meal preparation (Note to readers: pizza and pork-n-beans aren't such a bad combination), late night cups of tea, and cheering me on.

And to my princess and prince, Kayla and Michael Jaden, thank you for sharing mommy with this book project. I know it seemed like an eternity (Kayla, you asked so many times!), but look! We did it. You two inspire me to laugh harder, play more, love incessantly, and to be the best person I can be. For that, I thank you both. You are my life's greatest joy.

Appendix

Alternative Medicine

Association of Accredited Naturopathic
  Medical Colleges (AANMC)
3201 New Mexico Ave. NW, Suite 350
Washington, DC 20016
866-538-2267
info@aanmc.org
www.aanmc.org

Alternative Medicine Foundation, Inc.
PO Box 60016
Potomac, MD 20859
301-340-1960

info@amfoundation.org
www.amfoundation.org

Queen Afua
106 Kingston Ave.
Brooklyn, NY 11213
718-221-Heal
info@queenafuaonline.com
www.queenafuaonline.com

Attorneys

American Academy of Estate Planning
  Attorneys

4365 Executive Drive, Suite 850
San Diego, CA 92121
800-846-1555
www.aaepa.com

National Bar Association
1225 11th St. NW
Washington, DC 20001
202-842-3900
www.nationalbar.org

The National Conference of Black
   Lawyers
116 W 111th St.
New York, NY 10027
866-266-5091
www.ncbl.org

The Association of Black Women Attorneys
847A 2nd Ave.
Box 305
New York, NY 10017
212-332-0748
www.geocities.com.abwagroup

Budgeting

Judy Lawrence. *The Budget Kit: The Common
   Cents Money Management Workbook.*
   Dearborn Trade. Chicago, 2004

Brown, Jesse B. *Pay Yourself First: The African
   American Guide to Financial Success and
   Security.* Wiley. New Jersey, 2001.

Bridgforth, Glinda. *Girl, Get Your Money
   Straight: A Sister's Guide to Healing Your Bank
   Account and Funding Your Dreams in 7 Simple
   Steps.* Broadway. New York, 2002.

Child Support

U.S. Department of Health and Human
   Services
Administration for Children and
   Families
370 L'Enfant Promenade SW
Washington, DC 20447
www.acf.dhhs.gov

Federal Office of Child Support
   Enforcement
www.ocse.org

Child Support Network
212 E. Osborn Rd. Suite 210
Phoenix, AZ 85012
800-398-0500
info@childsupport.com
www.childsupport.com

National Coalition for Child Support
   Options
945 McKinney #414
Houston, TX 77002
866-244-1946
www.childsupportoptions.org

Childbirth Classes/Alternative Birthing Techniques

International Childbirth Education
   Association
952-854-8660
Info@icea.org

Lamaze International
800-368-4404
www.lamaze-childbirth.com

American Academy of Husband-
   Coached Childbirth
800-423-2397
In California: 800-422-4784
www.bradleybirth.com

Academy of Certified Birth Educators
   and Labor Support Professionals
800-444-8223
www.acbe.com

College Savings

U.S. Department of Education
800-USA-LEARN
www.ed.gov

College Savings Plan Network
2760 Research Park Dr.
Lexington, KY 40511
877-CSPN4YOU
www.collegesavings.org

Upromise Inc.
117 Kendrick St. Suite 200
Needham, MA 02494
888-434-9111
www.upromise.com

Debt Counseling

Consumer Debt Counseling
1300 Hampton Ave.
St. Louis, MO 63139
800-9-NO-DEBT
www.cccsstl.org

Consumer Credit Counseling Service
   (CCCS) a nonprofit service
800-873-2227
www.ccsintl.org

Dentists

American Dental Association
211 East Chicago Ave.
Chicago, IL 60611-2678
312-440-2500
www.ada.org

American Association of Dentists
330 S. Wells St. #1110
Chicago, IL 60606
800-920-2293
www.womandentists.org

Depression

American Psychiatric Association
1000 Wilson Blvd., Suite 1825
Arlington, VA 22209-3901
888-35-PSYCH (357-7924)
www.psych.org

American Psychological Association
750 First St. NE
Washington, DC 20022-4242
800-374-2721
www.apa.org

National Women's Health Information
  Center
8850 Arlington Blvd., Suite 300
Fairfax, VA 22031
800-994 WOMEN
www.4woman.gov

Diabetes

American Diabetes Association
1701 N. Beauregard St.
Alexandria, VA 22311
800-DIABETES
AskADA@diabetes.org
www.diabetes.org

National Institute of Diabetes &
  Digestive & Kidney Diseases
Office of Communications and Public
  Liaisons
NIDDK, NIH
Bethesda, MD 20892-2560
301-496-3583
www.niddk.nih.gov

Disability

Social Security Online
Social Security Administration
Office of Public Inquiries
6401 Security Blvd.
Baltimore, MD 21235
800-772-1213
www.ssa.gov

Disability Insurance Center
42 Ladd St., 2nd Floor
East Greenwich, RI 02818
www.disability-insurance-center.com

Discrimination During Pregnancy

AFSCME, Women's Rights Department
1625 L St. NW
Washington, DC 20036
202-429-5090
www.afscme.org.wrkplace/wrfaq06.htm

University of Michigan Health System
Smart Moms, Healthy Babies
1500 E. Medical Center Dr.

Ann Arbor, MI 48109
734-936-4000
www.med.umich.edu/obgyn/smartmoms

Gregory, Raymond F. *Women and Workplace Discrimination: Overcoming Barriers to Gender Equality*. Rutgers University Press. New Jersey, 2003.

Fibroids

National Uterine Fibroids Foundation
PO Box 9688
Colorado Springs, CO 80923-0688
719-633-3454
www.nuff.org

Brown, Monique R. *It's A Sistah Thing: A Guide to Understanding and Dealing with Fibroids for African American Women*. Kensington Publishing Corporation, New York, 2002.
www.nlm.nih.gov/medlineplus

Center for Uterine Fibroids
Brigham and Women's Hospital
Department of Obstetrics/Gynecology and Pathology
623 Thorn Building
20 Shattuck St.
Boston, MA 02115
(800) 722-5520 (x80081)
www.fibroids.net

Financial Planners/Investment Advisers

Financial Planning Association
1615 L St. NW, Suite 650
Washington, DC 20036-5606
800-322-4237
www.fpanet.org

Certified Financial Planner Board of Standards, Inc.
1670 Broadway, Suite 600
Denver, CO 80202-4809
303-830-7500
www.cfp.net

The North American Securities Administrators Association
750 First Street, N.E.
Suite 1140
Washington, DC 20002
202-739-0700
www.nasaa.org

National Association of Securities Dealers
9509 Key West Ave
Rockville, MD 20850
301-590-6500
www.nasd.com

NASD Broker Check Hotline
800-289-9999

Freelance Work/ Business Opportunities

Freelance Work Exchange
350 Bay St., Suite 276
San Francisco, CA 94133
415-358-4243
www.freelanceworkexchange.com

Sologig
333 Research Court Suite 200
Norcross, GA 30092
www.sologig.com

FreelanceMom.com
7 Hemlock Drive
Woodstock Valley, CT 06282
www.freelancemom.com

Federal Business Opportunities
877-472-3779
fbo.support@gsa.gov
www.fedbizopps.gov

United States Small Business
   Administration
409 Third St. SW
Washington, DC 20416
800 U ASK-SBA
www.sba.gov

Genetic Testing

The Genetics and Public Policy Center
1717 Massachusetts Avenue NW,
   Suite 530
Washington, DC 20036
202-663-5971
www.dnapolicy.org

Gene Tests
9725 Third Ave. NE, Suite 602
Seattle, WA 98115
206-616-4033
www.genetests.org

Health

Black Women's Health Project/Black
   Women's Health Imperative
600 Pennsylvania Avenue. S.E.,
   Suite 310
Washington, DC 20003
202-548-4000
www.blackwomenshealth.org

National Healthy Mothers, Healthy
   Babies Coalition
121 North Washington St., Suite 300
Alexandria, VA 22314
703-836-6110
www.hmhb.org

National Institute of Health
9000 Rockville Pike
Bethesda, MD 20892

301-496-4000
NIHinfo@od.nih.gov
www.nih.gov

National Women's Health Resource
    Center
157 Broad St., Suite 315
Red-Bank, NJ 07701
877-986-9472
info@healthywomen.org
www.wealthtywomen.org

HELLP/Preeclampsia

The HELLP Syndrome Society
www.hellpsyndrome.org

Preeclampsia Foundation
Administrative Office
5945 Maple Lane, Suite 101
Minnetonka, MN 55345-6427
800-665-9341
Info@preeclampsia.com
www.preeclampsia.org

HIV/AIDS

Black Women's Health
www.blackwomenshealth.com

AIDS.ORG
7985 Santa Monica Blvd. #99
West Hollywood, CA 90046
www.aids.org

AIDS Info
PO Box 6303
Rockville, MD 20849-6303
800 HIV 0440
http.//aidsinfo.nih.gov/live help

Household Help

Merry Maids
800-637-7962
www.merrymaids.com

The ServiceMaster Company
3250 Lacey Rd., Suite 600
Downers Grove, IL 60515
866-782-6787
www.servicemaster.com

GTM Household Employment Experts
7 Halfmoon Executive Park Drive
Clifton Park, NY 12065
888-4EASYPAY
www.gtmassociates.com

Radke, Linda F. *Nannies, Maids & More: The
    Complete Guide for Hiring Household Help.*
    Five Star Publications.
    Chandler, AZ 2000.

Hypertension

Pulmonary Hypertension Association
850 Sligo Ave., Suite 800
Silver Spring, MD 20910
800-748-7274

310-565-300
Fax 301-565-3994
www.phassociation.org

American Heart Association
National Center
7272 Greenville Ave.
Dallas, TX 75231
800-242-8721
www.americanheart.org

American Society of Hypertension, Inc.
148 Madison Ave., 5th Floor
New York, NY 10016
212-696-9099
www.ash-us.org

HypnoBirthing

HypnoBirthing Institute
PO Box 810
Epsom, NH 03234
877-798-3286
www.hypnobirthing.com

Mongan, Marie F. *HypnoBirthing: A Celebration of Life*. Health Communications Deerfield Beach, FL, 2005.

Insurance

Life and Health Insurance
Foundation for Education
2175 K St. NW, Suite 250

Washington, DC 20037
202-464-5000 x110
www.life-line.org

INSURANCE.COM
29001 Solon Rd.
Solon, OH 44139
866-533-0227
feedback@insurance.com
www.insurance.com

Esurance
747 Front St.
San Francisco, CA 94111
800-ESURANCE
800-378-7262
www.esurance.com

Insure.com
8205 S. Cass Avenue, Suite 102
Darien, IL 60561
800-556-9393
www.insure.com

Loss

SHARE Pregnancy & Infant Loss Support, Inc.
National SHARE Office
St. Joseph Hospital Center
300 First Capital Dr.
St. Charles, MO 63301-2893
800-821-6819
636-947-6164
www.nationalshareoffice.com

Center for Loss and Life Transitions
3735 Broken Bow Road
Fort Collins, CO 80526
970-226-6050
www.centerforloss.com

Grief Loss & Recovery
Joanne Glasspoole
PO Box 581277
Minneapolis, MN 55458-1277
800-211-1202 ×14436
www.grieflossrecovery.com

Lupus

Lupus Foundation of America, Inc.
2000 L St. NW, Suite 710
Washington, DC 20036
202-349-1155
www.lupus.org

U.S. National Library of Medicine and
    the National Institute Of Health
9000 Rockville Pike
Bethesda, MD 20892
301-496-4000
www.nlm.nih.gov/medlineplus

National Women's Health Information
    Center
8550 Arlington Blvd., Suite 300
Fairfax, VA 22031
800-994-Women
www.4woman.gov

Maternity Clothes

Professional Expectations
8971-B Metcalf
Overland Park KS 66212
888-381-7272
www.maternityleasing.com

Maternity Mall
456 N. 5th St.
Philadelphia, PA 19123
800-4mom2be
www.maternitymall.com

Maternity Leave

Work Options
Pat Katepoo, RD
WorkOption.com
47-370 Mawaena St
Kaneohe, HI 96744-4721
808-531-9939
www.workoptions.com

National Network for Child Care
Iowa State University Extension
1094 LeBaron Hall
Ames, IA 50001
www.nncc.org

Men

Hamer, Jennifer. *What It Means to Be Daddy: Fatherhood for Black Men Living Away from Their Children.* Columbia University Press. New York, 2001.

Taylor, Kristin Clark. *Black Fathers: A Call for Healing.* Doubleday. Garden City, New York, 2003.

Vanzant, Iyanla. *The Spirit of a Man.*

100 Black Men of America, Inc.
141 Auburn Ave.
Atlanta, GA 30303
800-598-3411
404-688-5100
www.100blackmen.org

Black Men in America.com
6503 Old Branch Ave., Suite 202
Temple Hills, MD 20748-2645
301-449-4335
www.blackmeninamerica.com

Mommy Support

Mocha Moms, Inc.
National Office
PO Box 1995
Upper Marlboro, MD 20773
nationaloffice@mochamoms.org

The Mommy & Me Association, Inc.
4100 W. Alameda
Burbank, CA 91505
818-955-5589
www.mommyandme.org

Mommy Too! Magazine
919 942-8024
info@mommytoo.co
www.mommytoo.com

Mortgage Brokers/Consultants

National Association of Mortgage Brokers
8201 Greensboro Dr., Suite 300
McLean, VA 22101
703-610 9009
www.namb.org

Nutrition

Food and Nutrition Information Center
Agricultural Research Service, USDA
National Agricultural Library, Rm. 105
10301 Baltimore Ave.
Beltsville, MD 20705-2351
301-504-5719
www.nal.usda.gov/fnic

The American Society for Nutritional Sciences
9650 Rockville Pike, Suite 4500
Bethesda, MD 20814

301-634-7050
sec@asns.org
www.asns.org

American Dietician Association
120 South Riverside Plaza, Suite 2000
Chicago, IL 60606-6995
800-877-1600
www.eatright.org

Older Moms

Midlife Mother Support
c/o Bonus Families
PO Box 1926
Discovery Bay, CA 94515
925-516-2681
www.midlifemother.com

Blackstone-Ford, Jann. *Midlife
Motherhood: A Woman-to-Woman Guide to
Pregnancy and Parenting*. St. Martin's
Press. New York, 2002.

Shanahan, M. Kelly. *Your Over-35 Week-
by-Week Pregnancy Guide*. Crown
Publishing Group. New York, 2001.

Ophthalmologists

American Academy of Ophthalmology
PO Box 7424
San Francisco, CA 94120-7424
415-561-8500
www.aao.org

The American Board of Ophthalmology
111 Presidential Blvd., Suite 241
Bala Cynwyd, PA 19004-1075
610-664-1175
www.abop.org

Overweight/Obesity

American Obesity Association
1250 24th St. NW, Suite 300
Washington, DC 20037
202-776-7711
www.obesity.org

Centers for Disease Control and
  Prevention
1600 Clifton Rd
Atlanta, GA 30333
800-311-3435
404-639-3534
www.cdc.gov/

Postabortion Support

Post Abortion Stress Syndrome
  Foundation
www.afterabortion.com

PASS Website
P.O. Box 2275
Glen Burnie, MD 21060
path@healingafterabortion.org
www.healingafterabortion.org

De Puy, Candace, and Dana Dovitch. *Healing Choice: Your Guide to Emotional Recovery after an Abortion*. DIANE Publishing. Collingdale, Pennsylvania, 2005.

Relationships

Miller, Denene, and Nick Chiles. *What Brothers Think, What Sistahs Know: The Real Deal on Love and Relationships*. HarperCollins. New York, 1999.

Black Women's Health
www.blackwomenshealth.com

1000 Questions for Couples
PO Box 1567
Cary NC 27512
919-462-0900
www.questionsforcouples.com

McGraw, Phillip C. *Relationship Rescue*. Hyperion. New York, 2001.

Sickle Cell

The Sickle Cell Information Center
PO Box 109
Grady Memorial Hospital
80 Jesse Hill Jr. Dr. SE
Atlanta, GA 30303
404-616-3572
aplatt@emory.edu
www.scinfo.org

Sickle Disease Association of America, Inc.
16 S. Calvert St., Suite 600
Baltimore, MD 21202
800-421-8453
www.sicklecelldisease.org

Platt, Allan F., and Alan Sacerdote. *Hope and Destiny: A Patient's and Parent's Guide to Sickle Cell Disease and Sickle Cell Trait*. Hilton Publishing. Munster, Indiana, 2001.

Single Mothers

Parents Without Partners, Inc.
1650 South Dixie Highway, Suite 510
Boca Raton, FL 33432
561-391-8833
www.parentswithoutpartners.org

Mattes, Jane. *Single Mothers by Choice: A Guidebook for Single Women Who Are Considering or Have Chosen Motherhood*. Random House. New York, 1997.

Skin Care

Taylor, Dr. Susan. *Brown Skin, Dr. Susan Taylor's Prescription for Flawless Skin, Hair, and Nails*. Amistad, New York.

The Skin of Color Center
Dept of Dermatology
St. Luke's–Roosevelt Hospital Center

1890 Amsterdam Avenue, Suite 11D
New York, NY 10025
800-753-3239

Carol's Daughter
Legacy Store
1 South Elliott Place
Fort Greene, NY
718-596-1862
www.carolsdaughter.com

Therapists/Psychiatrists/Psychologists

African American Therapists
www.africanamericantherapists.com

American Psychiatric Association
1000 Wilson Blvd., Suite 1825
Arlington, VA 22209-3901
703-907-7300
apa@psych.org
www.psych.org

The Association of Black Psychologists
PO Box 55999
Washington, DC 20040-5999
202-722-0808
office@abpsi.org
www.abpsi.org

Twins

National Organization of Mothers of
    Twins Clubs, Inc.
248-231-4480
877-540-2200
www.nomotc.org

The Twins Foundation
PO BOX 6043
Providence, RI 02940-6043
401-751-TWIN
www.twinsfoundation.com

CSMB
Center for the Study of Multiples
333 East Superior St., Suite 464
Chicago, IL 60611
312-695-1677
www.multiplbirth.com

Lyons, Elizabeth. *Ready or Not . . . Here We
    Come! The Real Experts' Cannot-Live-Without
    Guide to the First Year with Twins*. Xlibris
    Corp. Philadelphia, PA, 2003.

Index

Abel-Bey, Geddis, 142–44, 146, 148–49, 151, 156, 159
abortion:
  coping with, 203
  grieving after, 200, 202–3
acid stomach, 10
acne, 26
acupuncture, 11
African American women:
  abortion and, 201
  buying power of, 259–62
  caring for others by, 168, 178–79
  cravings in pregnancy of, 94–95
  depression and, 189–96

as fashion innovators, 219
media stereotypes and, 166
medical conditions of, 141–64
myths about, 5, 172
preterm labor of, 5
racism and, 165, 170–71, 174–76, 260–61
in slave communities, 4–5, 168, 171–72
spirituality of, 173, 178, 201, 203
Strong Black Woman (SBW) syndrome and, 167–68, 169, 172–74, 190
twin births of, 123

unplanned pregnancies of, 197
weight gain in, 9
African American Women's Voices Project, 166–67
African tribal traditions, 84, 94–95
age thirty-five and over:
  birth defects at, 130–33
  fears and risks at, 129–33
  personal comments on, 135
  postponing pregnancy at, 127–29
AIDS, see HIV/AIDS
Alabama, 95
alcohol intake, 145, 193

alpha-fetoprotein (AFP)
blood test, 148–49
Alzheimer's disease, 27
A. M. Best & Co., 266
American Cancer Society,
150
American College of
Obstetrics and
Gynecology, 6, 157
American Morning (TV show),
126
amniocentesis, 130–32,
163
amniotic fluid, 47, 127,
130–31, 149, 161
amniotic sac, 90, 125, 131
anal fissures, 17
Anderson, Pamela, 11, 230
Angela, 30
Angelou, Maya, 5
Ann, 131
antidepressants, 196
antihistamines, 244
anti-Ro antibodies, 153–54
Antwone Fisher (film), 138
Any Given Sunday (film), 214
appearance and morale,
66–67, 103–4, 115,
241–42
Aquaphor, 243
Ariel, 11
Arin, 33, 184–85
aromatherapy, 177
Audrey (Illinois), 89
Audrey (South Carolina),
87
autoantibodies, 153
Aveeno Oatmeal Bath, 244
Aveeno Positively Radiant,
243
AZT, *see* ZDV

Babies R Us, 68
BabyGap, 284
baby Guess!, 284
BabyMint, 279
Baby Phat, 220, 237, 239
BabyPlus, 138
baby showers, 281
Badu, Erykah, 11
Baldwin, Adam, 212–13
Baldwin, Blair, 212
Baldwin, Phyllis, 204,
212–13
Banana Republic, 220
Banks, Tyra, 11
Barbara, 192
Barney's Procreation, 218
Bebe, 220
Bella Mama's Belly Oil,
244
Benadryl, 244
Berry, Halle, 220, 249
BET, 8, 260
Bible, 168, 173
birth defects, 130–33, 149,
152
birthmarks, 88
*Black Pearls: Daily Meditations,
Affirmations and Inspirations for
African Americans* (Copage),
183
Blige, Mary J., 220
blood platelets, 206
blood sugar levels,
147–49
blurred vision, 25–26
BMI (body mass index),
150–51
body changes, 7–9
in first trimester, 44–46
in second pregnancy,
255–56

in second trimester,
55–56
in third trimester, 63–66
body image, 7–9, 33–37
body mass index (BMI),
150–51
Braxton-Hicks contractions,
64, 256
breast-feeding, 12, 88, 133,
198
breasts:
changes in, 11–12, 55
fungal infection and,
244
myths about, 87–88
Brianna, 120
Bridget, 284
Brooks Brothers, 220
*Brown Skin: Dr Taylor's Prescription
for Flawless Skin, Hair and Nails*
(Taylor), 242–43
Brown Sugar (film), 77
"Buck Naked and Beautiful"
(Mattox), 33–37
Bureau of Child Welfare,
U.S., 68
Bureau of the Census, U.S.,
261
Bush, Laura, 136
buttocks, changes in, 12

California, 61
car insurance, 273
Carlise (Illinois), 194
Carlise (New Jersey), 56
Carlos, 273
Carroll, Diahann, 220
castor oil, myths about,
89–90
Cedric the Entertainer,
110–12

Centers for Disease Control and Prevention (CDC), 5, 130, 147, 155–57, 197
cephalopelvic disproportion, 80
cervical weakness (incompetent cervix), 213
cervix, 64, 124, 131, 143–44, 213
cesarean birth, *see* C-sections
Cetaphil Antibacterial Soap, 243, 246
Cetaphil lotion, 249
Chantal, 58
Charisse, 7–8
chemical hair treatments, 85–87, 246–47
Cherita, 135
Chicago, Ill., 50
chicken pox, 48
childbirth classes, 62, 255
child care costs, 278
Child Support Enforcement office, 122
chorionic villius sampling (CVS), 131–32
chronic or serious illness, 192
Cinda, 202–3
Civil Rights Act of 1964, 61
clumsiness, 25–26, 56
CNN, 126, 180
Cochran, Johnny, 122
Cocoon (film), 17
cold remedies, 19
Colleen, 110
college funds, 278–80
Colorado, 197
Columbia University, 119, 262

compulsive spending, 285
conspicuous consumption, 260, 269
constipation, 16–17, 126
Consumer Federation of America, 260
contractions:
    Braxton-Hicks, 64, 256
    see also labor
Copage, Eric V., 183
Cora, 27, 102
Costco, 284
counseling, 121, 200, 210
CoverMark, 245
cravings, 28–29, 88, 94–95
Creative Nails Solar Oil, 249
credit card debt, 276–78
C-sections, 63, 69, 127, 150, 206, 252
    at age thirty-five and over, 130
    fibroids and, 145
    HIV and, 157
    Katrina Ruiz on, 80–81
    Lorna Kyle on, 110–12
    myths about, 92–93
    overweight/obesity and, 152
    placenta previa and, 114
    sickle cell disease and, 160–61
CVS (chorionic villius sampling), 131–32
Cynthia, 32

Daisy Dukes, 228–29
Damon, 105–6
Dandridge, Dorothy, 220
Darcelle, 135
Davia, 237
Debbi, 258

Debbie, 76, 135, 162, 272–73
Debra, 258
Debtors Anonymous, 285
deep breathing technique, 182
dehydration, 56, 160, 275
Deidre, 101
Denise, 18, 225, 236, 257
depilatories, avoidance of, 246
depression, 172
    after abortion, 202–3
    African American women and, 189–91
    coping with, 194–96
    possible causes of, 192
    postpartum, 193
    symptoms of, 191–92
    unplanned pregnancy and, 210–11
DermaBlend, 245
diabetes, 147–50
    managing of, 148–49
    risks from, 149–50
Diane (California), 38
Diane (New York), 237
Diane (South Carolina), 14
Dianne, 198–99
Dianne (New Jersey), 134
diet, *see* eating healthfully
dietary supplements, 18
digestion, 10, 15–16, 126
disability insurance, 268
dizzy spells, 10, 25–26
Donna, 135
Doppler sound-wave stethoscope, 47
Dove, 243
Down's syndrome, 130–33

"Drano test," 91
dreams, 27–28
Dr. Phil, 190
drug use, illegal, 193
Duo from JCPenney, 218
durable power of attorney,
    282–83

eating healthfully, 6–7,
    124–25, 146, 151, 254
Ebanks, Michelle, 67,
    161–64
ectopic pregnancy, 204
Eddie, 108
Egypt, 218
Elizabeth, 236
Elliott, Missy, 220
embryos, 46–47
Emory University, 174
emotions, 22
    after abortion, 202
    in the first trimester,
        44–46
    and hormone levels, 27
Employee Assistance
    programs, 195–96
epidurals, 62, 69, 80–81,
    137, 139
Equal Employment
    Opportunity Commission,
    61
Erica, 75, 205–8, 210
Escada, 220
Essence Communication
    Partners, 161
Essence magazine, 67, 161–62
Esther, 32
estrogen levels, 143–44
Eucerin lotion, 249
Eucerin Plus, 243
Eve, 220

exercise programs, 45–46,
    139
Express, 220, 225
Ezeilo, Angelou, 6–7

families:
    grieving in, 186–87
    pregnancy loss in, 205
    pregnancy myths in,
        83–85
    second pregnancies and,
        253
    sharing the news with, 38
    and the single mother,
        119–20
    stress in, 184–85
Family Law Code, 122
fetal cardiac echo, 155
fetal development:
    detecting gender and, 55
    in first trimester, 46–47
    nuchal translucency and,
        132
    in second trimester, 57
    testing of, 148–49, 155
    in third trimester, 69–70
fetal growth restriction,
    125–26, 147
fetal movements, 57, 199,
    256
fetal testing, 155, 160
fibroids, 143–45
    risks from, 144–45
financial planning, 105,
    121–22
    African American buying
        power, 259–62
    baby showers in, 281
    budget worksheet in,
        286–88
    car insurance in, 273

cash flow analysis in,
    268–71
college funds in, 278–80
cost-cutting and saving in,
    272–76, 278
credit card debt in,
    276–78, 284–85
freelancing and, 263
housing costs and, 274–75
life insurance in, 266–68
refinancing a mortgage in,
    272–73
self-evaluation in,
    264–66, 268, 275,
    280
single mothers and,
    121–22
for stay-at-home mothers,
    262–65
talking with partners in,
    266, 271, 284
wills and trusts in,
    281–83
your child's future in, 264
first trimester:
    body changes in, 44–46
    chemical hair treatments
        in, 246
    fetal development in,
        46–47
    financial planning in,
        265–75
    maternity clothes in,
        222–23
    sexual relations in, 23
    testing in, 131
    travel in, 49–50
    weight gain in, 9
    workplace conditions in,
        47–53
Fitzgerald, Ella, 220

Fleming, Denise, 28, 53, 62, 69
folic acid levels, 132, 152, 197
Food Network, 28
401(K) funds, 261, 276, 282
friends, 109
    changing relationships with, 97–104
    importance of, 97, 101–2
    pregnancy loss and, 205
    second pregnancy and, 253
    sharing the news with, 38–39
    single mother and, 120–21
    socializing with, 99
    too much information and, 101
Friends (TV show), 123
"From Fab to Flab: My Pregnancy Journey" (Mischel-Wilson), 112–15
FUBU, 220
funerals, attendance at, 91–92
Fuqua, Antoine, 214
Fuqua, Asia, 215
Fuqua, Lela Rochon, 204, 214–16

Gallup poll, 167
Gap, 218
gas, 15
gender detection, 55, 90–91
genetic testing, 131–33
geophagy (pica), 94–95
German measles, 48
gestational diabetes, 130
Ghana, 218
girlfriends, see friends

glands of Montgomery, 55
glucose levels, 147–48
Golden Globe awards, 214
Good Times (TV show), 261
Grace, 206–8
graduated compression stockings, 20
Great Britain, 92–93, 117
grief counselors, 210
grieving:
    after abortion, 200, 202–3
    Karen Shaw on, 186–87
    after pregnancy loss, 204–5, 208–9
guilt feelings, 191–92, 195, 197, 201–2, 253–54
gums, 14, 55

hair:
    change in texture of, 247
    chemical treatments for, 85–87, 246–47
    excessive perspiration and, 248
    growth/loss of, 13–14
    low-maintenance style and, 248–49
Harlem, New York, 119
Harlem Nights (film), 214
Harrison, Roderick, 260
Harvard University, 280
Hawaii, 61
headaches, 56
Health Department, U.S., 153
HELLP syndrome, 206
hematologists, 159
hemorrhoids, 17
high blood pressure, 149, 172

managing of, 146
risks from, 147, 152, 206
high-risk pregnancy obstetrician, see perinatologists
hirsutism, pregnancy-induced, 13–14, 245–46
HIV/AIDS:
    and African American women, 155–56, 172
    managing of, 156–57
    risks from, 157
HIV-infected babies, 157
holistic and alternative medicine, 187
Home Depot, 30
home pregnancy tests, 113
hormone levels, 193
    in constipation, 16
    in depression, 190
    in diabetes, 148
    in emotions, 27
    fibroids and, 143
    gums and, 14
    in hair growth and loss, 13–14
    in headaches, 56
    in morning sickness, 10
    in skin problems, 242–43, 245
    in stress, 169
    in twin births, 127
    in urination, 24–25
Horne, Lena, 220
hospital care, pregnancy loss and, 204–8
human chorionic gonadotropin (hCG), 45
human immunodeficiency virus (HIV), 155–57
Hurston, Zora Neale, 5

hyperpigmentation, 243
hypertension:
    pregnancy-induced, 130
    see also high blood pressure
hypervigilancc, 168
hypno-birthing, 139
Hypnotiq, 88
hypoglycemia, 148

Illinois, 197
incontinence, postlabor
    stress, 130
individual retirement
    accounts (IRAs), 261, 282
inducing labor, 150, 152
infant deaths, 5, 169–70,
    204
inferior vena cava, 20
insomnia, 65–66
insulin, 147–49
insurance, 39, 61–62
    car, 273
    life, 121, 266–68
    temporary disability,
        61–62
Internet resources, 121, 129,
    225, 229, 273, 279
IRAs (individual retirement
    accounts), 261, 282
Ireland, 48
Isabel, 253
Ivy, 32, 74, 258
Iyanla, 6

Jackson, Andrea M.,
    142–44, 146, 148, 151–52,
    154–55, 157–59
Jackson, Gail N., 142,
    144–46, 149, 151–52, 159
Jamal, 131
James, 105

Jamilia, 175
Janaris, 75
Janeen, 41
Janelle, 263
Japanese Weekend, 218
Jasmin, 76
jaundice, 150
Jeanne, 32
Jesus Christ, 173, 190
Jill, 273
Jim Crow laws, 190
Joint Center for Political
    and Economic Studies,
    260
Jones, Charisse, 166, 173
Jones, Jacqueline, 171–72
Joyce, 45, 91

Kaia, 13–14
Kareen, 22
Katrice, 52–53
Kegel exercises, 21, 130
Keishawn, 124
Keiva, 102
Kent State University, 176
Kenya, 277–78
Kevin, 207–8
Keys, Alicia, 220
Kiana, 60
Kim, 24
Kimbro, Dennis, 265–66
Knowles, Beyoncé, 8, 220
Kodjoe, Boris, 77–79
Kush, 218
Kyle, Lorna, 110–12

LaBelle, Patti, 220
labor, 72–73
    anxiety during, 203
    hormone level and, 127
    inducing of, 74, 150, 152

myths about, 89–90
    pain management, 62,
        69
    personal comments on,
        73–74
    planning for, 63, 69
    preterm, 5, 14, 23, 47,
        124, 144–45, 149, 159
Labor of Love, Labor of Sorrow:
    Black Women, Work, and the
    Family from Slavery to the
    Present (Jones), 171–72
Lamar, 272–73
Latimore, Kenny, 29
Laura, 131
Lauren, 76
Lavania, 256
Lee, Sophie Tei-Naaki, 77
leg cramps, 18
Leila, 89
leucorrhea, 20–21
Lever 2000, 244
life insurance, 121,
    266–68
light therapy, 183, 196
Lil' Kim, 229
linea nigra, 20
Lisa (Georgia), 41
Lisa (Buffalo, N.Y.), 133
Lisa (New York, N.Y.), 58
Lisa (White Plains, N.Y.),
    74–76
"Little Boy Lost" (Rochon),
    214–16
Liz Lange, 218, 223, 237
LL Cool J, 107
London, England, 60, 117
Lorraine, 28, 31, 33,
    74, 76
Los Angeles Times, 201
LouAnn, 134

low-birth-weight babies, 5,
    14, 47, 124, 126, 145, 152,
    161, 169–70, 193
lupus, 153–55
    managing of, 154–55
    risks from, 155
Lupus Foundation of
    America, 153
Lynette, 31–32

Maat'ra, Djehuty, 79
McMillan, Terry, 128
macrosomia, 149
Maisha, 134
Mali, 218–19
March of Dimes, 5, 157
March of Dimes Task Force
    on Nutrition and Optimal
    Human Development, 152
Mary, 11
"mask of pregnancy"
    (melasma), 26, 244–45
maternal anemia, 125
maternity clothes:
    accessories for, 221,
        230–31
    casual wear in, 227
    for every body type,
        234–36
    in first trimester, 222–23
    Kimora Lee Simmons on,
        237–39
    personal comments on,
        236–37
    and pregnancy style,
        217–22, 234–36
    renting careerwear for,
        225, 229
    in second trimester,
        223–24
    and shoes, 231

for special occasions,
    229–30
for summertime, 228–29
ten things you need in,
    233–34
in third trimester, 231–33
for work, 224–27
maternity leave, 39, 59, 128,
    264, 271
Mattox, Kuae Kelch, 7, 31,
    33–37, 74, 109
meconium, 89–90
media stereotypes, 166, 175
Medicaid, 169
medical conditions:
    diabetes, 147–50
    fibroids, 143–45
    high blood pressure,
        145–47, 206
    HIV/AIDS, 155–57
    lupus, 153–55
    overweight/obesity,
        150–53
    sickle cell disease, 158–61
melasma ("mask of
    pregnancy"), 26, 244 45
memory decline, 26–27, 54
Meredith, 202
Michigan, University of,
    Depression Center
    Women's Mood Disorders
    Program at, 193
Millner, Denene, 6
Mimi Maternity, 218
miscarriage, 50, 54, 204
    at age thirty-five and over,
        130, 163
    diabetes and, 149
    fibroids and, 144
    lupus and, 154–55
    sexual relations and, 23

sickle cell disease, 160–61
    test-related, 131
    working conditions and,
        86–87, 171
Mischelle, 88
Mischel-Wilson, Jennifer,
    112–15
Mocha Moms, 187
moles and skin tags, 26,
    245
moodiness, 22, 44
"More Than the Blues"
    (Whitfield), 210–12
morning sickness, 9–11, 52,
    125–26, 160, 162
mortgage refinancing,
    272–73
Motherhood Maternity,
    218
"Motherless Child,
    Pregnancy After the Loss
    of My Mom" (Shaw),
    186–87
Mozart, Wolfgang Amadeus,
    57
music and brain
    development, 57
Musiq Soulchild, 29
Mya (Louisiana), 177
Mya (Virginia), 75
myomectomy, 63

nails, 14, 249
Nanette, 222
Naomi, 103
nasal congestion, 18–19
National Black Women's
    Health Project, 121, 196
National Institute of Child
    Health and Human
    Development, 157

National Institute of
    Diabetes and Digestive and
    Kidney Diseases
    (NIDDK), 148
National Mental Health
    Association, 191
National Survey of Family
    Growth, 196–97
natural childbirth, 72–73
nausea, 10–11, 54, 144
navels, 65
NBC News, 35
Neal-Barnett, Angela,
    176–77, 178, 180
neonatal death, 204
neonatal lupus, 154
"nesting," 68–69
neural tube defects, 148–49,
    152, 197
Neutrogena Facial Cleanser,
    246
Neutrogena lotion, 249
New Jersey, 61
New York, 61
New York City, 49, 228, 274
New York University (NYU),
    262
Nicole, 225
Nigeria, 123
nuchal translucency, 132
nutritionists, 146, 151

O'Brien, Soledad, 126,
    136–37, 180, 195
obstetrician, high-risk
    pregnancy, see
    perinatologists
Ohio State University, 191
Old Navy, 218, 223
orgasms, 22–23
overweight/obesity, 150–53

managing of, 151–52
risks from, 151–53

pain management, 69
Pam, 134
Pamela, 257
Parker, Nicole, 77–79
partners, 104–5, 107
    emotional dependence on,
        54
    fear of change and, 105–6
    financial concerns of, 105,
        253, 266, 271, 284
    personal comments on,
        40–41, 110
    in pregnancy loss, 205,
        207–8, 210
    in second pregnancies,
        253
    sharing the news with,
        40–41
    and the single mother,
        121–22
    stress and, 177–78
    in unplanned pregnancies,
        198–99, 211
PAS (postabortion
    syndrome), 201–2
Patrice, 16
Patricia, 27
Pea in the Pod, 218
Pell Grants, 280
perinatologists, 146, 154,
    156, 159
periodontal disease, 14
perspiration, excessive, 244,
    248
Phat Farm, 220
Phyllis, 40, 98, 109, 180,
    209
piles, see hemorrhoids

placenta, 57, 93, 125, 131,
    144–45, 155
placental abruption, 125,
    147, 154
placenta previa, 114, 129
Plato, 95
PMS (premenstrual
    syndrome), 27, 44, 183
Polo by Ralph Lauren, 284
postabortion help center,
    203
postabortion syndrome
    (PAS), 201–2
postpartum depression, 193
postpartum hemorrhage,
    145
Pre-and Perinatal Psychology
    Journal, 202–3
preeclampsia, 125, 129, 147,
    149, 152, 155, 161, 206
pregnancy:
    after abortion, 200–203
    at age thirty-five and over,
        127–33
    announcing of, 38–41,
        54, 60, 255–56
    and being your own health
        advocate, 161–64
    common myths about,
        83–95
    depression in, 189–96
    emotions in, 22, 27, 44,
        199–200
    financial planning in,
        259–88
    hair, skin, and nail
        problems in, 241–49
    Jennifer Mischel-Wilson
        on, 112–15
    managing stress in,
        165–87

maternity clothes and,
217–39
medical conditions among
African American
women in, 141–64
personal comments on,
31–33, 75–76, 133–35
preparing for, 3–9,
29–33, 38–41
relationships and, 97–115
second, 251–58
and the single mother,
117–22
slavery and, 4–5, 171–72
in summertime,
228–29
trimester-by-trimester
guide to, 43–71
twins and, 123–27
unplanned, 107–8, 117,
196–200, 210–12
workplace conditions and,
47–49
"pregnancy brain," 27, 54
pregnancy depression,
189–96
Pregnancy Discrimination
Act of 1978, 61
pregnancy gingivitis, 14
pregnancy loss:
coping with, 208–10
Erica on, 206–8, 210
funeral or memorial
services in, 208–9
grieving in, 204–5,
208–9
Lela Rochon on, 214–16
partners and, 205,
207–8, 210
Phyllis Baldwin on,
212–13

pregnancy myths:
attending funerals, 91–92
castor oil, 89–90
chemical hair treatments,
85–87
cravings, 88, 94–95
gender detection, 90–91
sexual relations, 24
sleeping positions, 93–94
small shoe size, 92–93
sore breast remedy, 87–88
umbilical cord
strangulation, 83–85
premature birth, 193
premature dilation, 124
premenstrual syndrome
(PMS), 27, 44, 183
prenatal group therapy,
108
prescription drug use, 194
preterm labor, 5, 14, 23, 47,
124, 144–45, 149, 159
private therapy, 196
problems:
at age thirty-five and over,
129–33
Braxton-Hicks
contractions, 64
clumsiness, 25–26, 56
constipation, 16
depression, 189–96
discomfort at work, 59–60
gas, 15
gum disease, 14, 55
headaches, 56
hemorrhoids, 17
leg cramps, 18
moodiness, 22, 44
morning sickness, 9–11,
52, 125
round ligament pain, 56

runny nose/nasal
congestion, 18–19
skin ailments, 26, 65
spider veins/varicose veins,
19–20
stretch marks, 15–16
swelling, 50, 66
third trimester, 64–66
twin pregnancies, 125–26
urination, 24–25
vaginal discharge, 20–21
vomiting, 23, 52, 54, 136,
144
Program for Research on
Anxiety Disorders among
African Americans, 176
prolapse, 129
Public Health Service, U.S.,
156
Puerto Rico, 62
pulmonary embolus, 152
Pumpkin Maternity, 218

Queen Afua, 78
"Queen of the C, The"
(Ruiz), 80–81

racism, 165–66, 170–71,
174–76, 260–61
Rajine, 107
Raquel, 25
Rashaun, 40
rashes, 16, 26, 65, 244
Reaganomics, 190
Reconstruction, 190
Reese, 257
relationships:
and depression, 195
with family, 38, 83–85,
119–20, 184–85
fear of change in, 105–6

relationships, continued
  financial concerns in, 105
  with girlfriends, 97–104
  with partners, 104–8
  sharing pregnancy details
    in, 101
  stress in, 107–8, 177–78,
    184–85
Remember the Titans (film),
  77
Renee, 134
respiratory distress
  syndrome, 150
rest, importance of, 53, 127,
  181
retinopathy, 148
revocable trusts, 283
Rhode Island, 62
Rochelle, 237
Rochon, Lela, *see* Fuqua,
  Lela Rochon
Rollins School of Public
  Health, 174–75
Ross, Diana, 128
round ligament pain, 56
Roxanne, 68
Ruiz, Katrina, 80–81
runny nose, 18–19

Sabrina, 261
Sacrament of the Sick, 206
Sacred Women (Afua), 78
salt intake, 145–46
Sandra (Alabama), 129
Sandra (New Jersey), 108
Sara, 46
SBW (Strong Black Woman
  syndrome), 167–68, 169,
  172–74, 190
Schalawn, 49, 102, 229
Sea-Bands, 10–11

Sean John, 220
second pregnancies, 251–53
  body changes in, 255–56
  emotional distance from,
    254–55
  personal comments on,
    257–58
second trimester, 163
  body changes in, 55–56
  chemical hair treatments
    in, 86
  fetal development in, 57
  fibroids in, 144
  financial planning in,
    275–80
  high blood pressure in,
    146
  leg cramps in, 18
  lupus in, 155
  maternity clothes in,
    223–24
  "pregnancy brain" in, 54
  sexual relations in, 23
  weight gain in, 9, 54–55
  and workplace conditions,
    58–62
sexism, 165–66, 170–71
sexual relations, 21–24, 56
  abstinence from, 23
  myths about, 24
  orgasms and, 22–23
Shakur, Tupac, 5
Shanice, 225
Sharpton, Al, 166
Shaun, 32
Shavonda, 134
Shaw, Karen, 186–87
Sheena, 94
Shelley, 271
Sherese, 102
Sherri, 177

Sheryl, 51, 76
"shifting," 166–67
*Shifting-The Double Lives of
  Black Women in America* (Jones
  and Shorter-Gooden),
  173
Shorter-Gooden, Kumea,
  166, 173
shortness of breath, 45, 126
shoulder distotia, 150
sickle cell disease, 158–61
  managing of, 159–60
  risks from, 160–61
SIDS (sudden infant death
  syndrome), 171
Simmons, Kimora Lee, 67,
  220, 221, 231, 237–39
Simmons, Russell, 237
Simone, Nina, 5
Simone (New York), 120
Simone (Ohio), 177–78
single mothers:
  and emotional stress,
    117–18
  facing disapproval by,
    118–21
  and legal matters, 122
  personal comments on,
    133–34
Sistah's Rules, The (Millner),
  6
Skin of Color Center, Saint
  Luke's-Roosevelt Hospital,
  242
skin problems:
  acne, 26, 242–43
  excessive perspiration, 244
  facial hair (hirsutism),
    245–46
  hyperpigmentation
    (darkening), 243–44

"mask of pregnancy" (melasma), 26, 244–45
moles, 245
rashes, 65, 244
slave communities, 4–5, 168, 171–72
sleeping positions, 93–94
socializing at work, 58–59
Sondra, 275
sonograms, 47–48, 55, 123, 149, 152
Soothe Your Nerves: A Black Woman's Guide to Understanding and Overcoming Anxiety, Panic and Fear (Neal-Barnett), 176–77
Sophia, 169
Soul Food (TV series), 77, 101
South African Medical Journal, 89
South Carolina, 119
spider veins, 19–20
spina bifida, 132, 152
spirituality, 173, 178, 200–201, 203
Stacey, 129
Stephanie (New York), 257
Stephanie (Washington D.C.), 86, 134
stillbirths, 149–50, 154–55, 161, 204
stress:
    in caring for others, 168, 178
    coping with, 51–53, 173–74, 176–77, 178–79, 181–85
    depression and, 191
    five ways to de-stress, 182–83

four ways to defuse drama, 184–85
in grieving, 186–87
identifying of, 169–70
physical responses to, 167–68
racism/sexism and, 165–66, 170–71, 174–76
in relationships, 107–8, 177–78, 184–85
"shifting" and, 166–67
single mothers and, 117–18
spirituality and, 173
in unplanned pregnancies, 197
unrealistic goals and, 180–81
at work, 51–53, 70–71, 170–71, 174–77
stretch marks, 15–16
Strong Black Woman (SBW) syndrome, 167–68, 169, 172–74, 190
sudden infant death syndrome (SIDS), 171
summer clothing tips, 228–29
sunscreens, 243, 245
support groups, 120–21, 124, 187, 196, 210
Suzanne, 58
swelling, 50, 66

Taco Bell, 28
Talbots, 220
Tamia, 125
Tamika, 105–6
Tamisha, 204–5
tampons, avoidance of, 20
Tanya, 75, 106
Target, 223, 237

Tarsha, 75
Taylor, Susan C., 242–49
temporary disability insurance, 61
Think and Grow Rich: A Black Choice (Kimbro), 266
third trimester:
    appearance and morale in, 66–67
    baby preparations in, 68–69
    body changes in, 63–66
    clumsiness in, 25–26
    fear of pain in, 62–63
    fetal development in, 69–70
    fetal tests in, 155, 160
    financial planning in, 280–84
    leg cramps in, 18
    maternity clothes in, 231–33
    weight gain in, 9
    and workplace conditions, 70–71
Tia, 27, 41
Tina, 27
tobacco use, 10, 49, 193
Tony, 106
Tonya, 94
toxemia, 206
Tracey, 10, 15
Tracey Reese, 220
Training Day (film), 214
travel, 49–50
triple-screen blood test, 132
TV Guide, 285
twins:
    emotional stress and, 123–24

twins, *continued*
  healthy eating and, 124–25
  importance of rest and, 127
  personal comments on, 134
  problems of, 125–27
  Soledad O'Brien on, 136–37
twin-to-twin transfusion syndrome, 126

ultrasound, 131–32, 155
umbilical cord, 83–85
underwear, 12–13, 21, 217
unplanned pregnancies, 107–8, 117
  African American women and, 197
  coping with, 199–200
  infant health and, 197–98
  Jeanne Whitfield on, 210–12
Upromise, 279–80
urinary tract infections, 146, 149, 160
urination, 24–25

vaginal discharge, 20–21
Vanessa, 51
varicose veins, 19–20, 126
vena cava, 93–94
vitamin E, 243
vomiting, 23, 52, 54, 136, 144
von Furstenberg, Diane, 226

Waiting to Exhale (film), 214
Walker, C. J., Madame, 241
Wal-Mart, 223
Warren, Barbara Jones, 191, 194–95
Web sites, 39, 267
"Weeping for Adam: Pregnancy After a Stillbirth" (Baldwin), 212–13
weight gain, 9, 54–55, 114, 127, 139, 151, 192
Wendy, 32
Wendy's, 252
West Africa, 94–95, 142
What Brothers Think, What Sistahs Know (Millner and Chiles), 6
What to Expect When You're Expecting, 194
"Whistle While You Work," 51
Whitfield, D'ondre, 138–39
Whitfield, Jeanne, 198, 210–12
Whitfield, Salli Richardson, 138–39
Why Do Fools Fall in Love? (film), 214
Winfrey, Oprah, 190
Women's Mood Disorders Program, University of Michigan Depression Center, 193
work:
  announcing pregnancy at, 39–40, 255–56
  benefits available at, 267
  coping with discomfort at, 59–60
  in first trimester, 47–49, 50–53
  maternity clothes for, 224–27
  personal comments on, 75–76
  pregnancy discrimination at, 60–62
  pregnancy loss and, 215
  racism/sexism at, 165–66, 174–76
  returning to, after childbirth, 262, 264–65, 277
  risks to pregnancy at, 49, 86–87
  in second trimester, 58
  socializing at, 58–59
  stress management at, 51–53, 70–71, 170, 174–77
  in third trimester, 70–71
World Trade Center, 162
Wright, Daria, 246–49

yeast infections, 244
Yoruba Oshogbo tribe, Nigeria, 123
Yvette (New York), 166
Yvette (Virginia), 109

ZDV (zidovudine) (AZT), 156
zygotes, 46